Empathy-Based Ethics

David Ian Jeffrey

Empathy-Based Ethics

A Way to Practice Humane Medicine

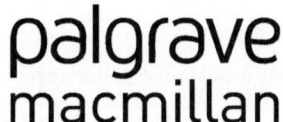

David Ian Jeffrey
Worcester, UK

ISBN 978-3-030-64803-9   ISBN 978-3-030-64804-6   (eBook)
https://doi.org/10.1007/978-3-030-64804-6

Cover illustration: © Harvey Loake

This Palgrave Macmillan imprint is published by the registered company Springer Nature
Switzerland AG
The registered company address is: Gewerbestrasse 11, 6330 Cham, Switzerland

To Pru

ACKNOWLEDGMENTS

I would like to thank my wife Pru for all her support and encouragement. I wish to thank Grace Jackson, Aishwarya Balachandar, Azarudeen Ahamed Sheriff and the publishing team at Palgrave Macmillan for their advice and help. I am grateful to the reviewers of my original book proposal for their wise feedback which has strengthened the arguments in the book. I have learned much about relating to patients from inspirational colleagues and teachers throughout my career including; Bill Astley, Lesley Dawson, Derek Doyle, Sean Elyan, Marie Fallon, Bobbie Farsides, Karen Forbes, Ken Jarrett, Rob Jarvis, Marilyn Kendall, Kathy Keogh, John Munro, Ray Owen. MR Rajagopal, Huw Richards, Michael Ross and Mike Whitfield. I am grateful to the many patients whose courage has taught me about coping with adversity.

CONTENTS

LIST OF FIGURES

CHAPTER 1

Introduction

Abstract There is concern that the patient-doctor relationship is damaged and medical practice is less humane. In an overview of the book, evidence of the dehumanisation of patients is discussed. Clarifying the nature of empathy, a first step towards humanising medical practice is followed by a broad relational model of empathy including virtues such as compassion, sympathy, kindness, generosity and humility. The process of empathy in the context of the patient-doctor relationship is examined. The aims and role of empathy are described before outlining the need for a different approach to medical ethics to enable humane medical care. Empathy-based ethics is a clinical approach, linked to both virtue ethics and care ethics, supplementing conventional bioethical principles. After examples of the approach in clinical practice, ways in which the empathy-based approach might be embedded in clinical practice, medical education and research are debated before looking to the future for empathy-based ethics.

Keywords Empathy-based ethics · Humane · Dehumanisation · Patient-doctor relationship

© The Author(s), under exclusive license to Springer Nature
Switzerland AG 2020
D. I. Jeffrey, *Empathy-Based Ethics*,
https://doi.org/10.1007/978-3-030-64804-6_1

INTRODUCTION

Ethics is the study of the moral way in which we should behave and interact with others. At its heart, ethics is concerned with relationships. The patient-doctor relationship is fundamental to the provision of high-quality medical care. Today, there is concern this core relationship is damaged, leading to a quality of care crisis, sometimes described as the dehumanisation of medicine (Haque and Waytz 2012; Marcum 2008; Montgomery 2006). The Francis Report detailed gross failings in patient care in the Mid Staffordshire NHS Foundation Trust (de Zulueta 2013b; Francis 2013; Haque and Waytz 2012; Jeffrey 2019). The report detailed instances of the dehumanisation of patients: uncaring staff attitudes, a failure to respect patients' dignity with a persistent neglect of patients' basic needs such as hygiene and nutrition (de Zulueta 2013b). Francis called for a change to a more patient-centred culture to ensure fundamental standards of care in the NHS. He reflected on 'appalling and unnecessary suffering', summarising five essential objectives, three involving the culture and communication within clinical care: compassionate caring, patient-centred leadership and openness (Francis 2013; Simpson and Morris 2014). Healthcare professionals and members of the public were shocked by the findings detailed in the report, resulting in a resurgence of interest to humanise medical care. The Chief Nursing Officer echoed Francis' concerns in her recommendation to nurses (Cummings and Bennett 2012).

Further evidence of a lack of humane care was provided in the Parliamentary Health Service Ombudsman's report: a lack of compassion and a failure to recognise the humanity of frail elderly patients (Parliamentary Health Service Ombudsman 2011):

> the action of individual staff described here add up to an ignominious failure to look beyond the patient's clinical condition and to respond to the social and emotional needs of the individual and their family (Parliamentary Health Service Ombudsman 2011).

The Parliamentary Health Service Ombudsman concluded that breaches of care were widespread and strongly recommended that the NHS should respond to the failings in care identified in her report.

Realistic Medicine, a report from the Chief Medical Officer, NHS Scotland, highlighted the need for a personalised approach to care and a change to shared decision-making (Calderwood 2016). Berwick argued for a paradigm change in health care in the USA, specifically to listen to the patients' concerns (Berwick 2016).

An underlying cause of the lack of humane care is the imbalance between the biomedical and psychosocial dimensions of medical practice (Marcum 2008). Scientific-technical, or biomedical, aspects of medical practice currently dominate patient care, while psychosocial elements are often neglected (Montgomery 2006). The biomedical model of practice simply reduces the patient to a physical body composed of parts, where the doctor's role is to identify and treat the diseased pieces using the latest technology and evidence-based research to cure the patient. A consequence of applying this model is that the patient becomes alienated from the doctor and feels as though they are treated as objects, i.e. dehumanised (Haque and Waytz 2012; Marcum 2008). Marcum maintains that the concept of a patient as a unique person disappears before the biomedical gaze (Marcum 2008). The emphasis on the 'objective', emotionally distant, biomedical model has eroded the patient-doctor relationship, contributing to the dehumanisation of medicine.

The humanisation of medicine involves redressing this imbalance. At the heart of humanising medicine lies empathy. To humanise is to 'make things less unpleasant for people, to show that someone has the qualities that are typical of a human, in a way that makes you more likely to feel sympathy for them' (Cambridge English Dictionary 2020). Patients want a feeling of connection with a doctor they know and trust (Derksen et al. 2013).

The concerns relating to the lack of humane medical care are compounded by a perception that medical students lose empathy as they progress through their undergraduate education (Hojat et al. 2009). However, recent research sheds doubt on these claims and suggests ways in which the student experience may be enhanced (Jeffrey 2019; Quince et al. 2016).

Chapter 2 begins by defining humane medicine and then describes the problem to be addressed by the book, a lack of humane care in medical practice or the dehumanisation of patients. Dehumanisation has been described in a number of ways—as detached concern, objectivity, distancing or the inhumanity of medicine (Halpern 2001; Mallia 2013; Weatherall 1994). Dehumanisation in medicine is defined, and its causes explored, reduced patient individuality and decreased patient autonomy, the biomedical-psychosocial imbalance, an empathy gap and moral distancing (Haque and Waytz 2012). There is a need to integrate evidence-based medicine and patient-centred medicine (Bensing 2000). The chapter concludes by advocating an innovative approach to address these issues, a relational form of clinical ethics with empathy at its core: empathy-based ethics (EBE).

Clarifying the nature of empathy is the first step towards human-ising medical practice. In Chapter 3, a broad relational model of empathy is described, addressing the ethical needs of patients, health-care professionals and the wider society. Empathy is a complex concept variously described as: feeling what another person feels, 'caring about others', imagining oneself in another's situation, having the capacity to grasp the content of other people's minds and a virtue in response to suffering (Batson 2011; Coplan and Goldie 2011). Empathy-based ethics provides an approach which promotes the humanisation of patients in medical practice and undergraduate medical education. The complexity of empathy is magnified by its relationship with other pro-social constructs such as sympathy and compassion (Jeffrey 2016).

In Chapter 4, the close relationships between empathy and sympathy, kindness, generosity and humility are explored. In particular, empathy and compassion are often muddled in the medical literature and in everyday speech, the differences between them are clarified. An argument is made for establishing empathy, rather than compassion, at the core of the relational ethical approach.

Chapter 5 explores the process of empathy in the context of the patient-doctor relationship. Empathy as a relational experience is profoundly affected by the context of the meeting between a patient and a doctor. The organisational culture, lack of time and stress may each influ-ence the process of empathy, which involves face-to-face contact between a patient and a doctor. The process of empathy involves a dynamic interplay between self-awareness, reflection, imagination, emotions and perspective taking. The next chapter discusses the importance of empathy in clinical practice.

Chapter 6 looks at the aims and role of empathy in clinical practice and in humanising medicine. Empathic relationships benefit both patients and their healthcare professionals. The benefits include patient satisfac-tion, health outcomes and the creation of trust (Mallia 2013). Empathy is instrumental in altruism and central in adopting a patient-orientated approach. Empathy's benefits to healthcare professionals include greater job satisfaction, better decision-making and protection against burnout (Kearney et al. 2009; Sturzu et al. 2019).

Chapter 7 examines the need for a different approach to medical ethics to complement the current judgemental models. Philosophers and ethicists have contributed to the discipline of theoretical bioethics, providing guidelines to address particular ethical dilemmas such as euthanasia, abortion or organ transplantation. Such ethical theories include deontology and utilitarianism and the four-principle approach. However, the four-principle approach: autonomy, beneficence, non-maleficence and justice, does not contribute to improving the patient experience. A fresh clinical ethical approach is needed if medical care is to be more humane. Empathy-based ethics is a clinical approach which supplements conventional ethical principlism and is linked to both virtue ethics and care ethics. In defining empathy-based ethics, related virtues such as humility, generosity, sympathy and kindness are explored. Care ethics is closely related to empathy-based ethics; therefore, the essential features and the limitations of care ethics are outlined in establishing a case for the empathy-based ethics approach (EBE). Critics of empathy point to its susceptibility to bias, exploring this supposed limitation of empathy strengthens the empathy-based ethical approach (Macnaughton 2009).

A new clinical ethical approach requires to be interrogated in difficult clinical situations. Chapter 8 examines the EBE approach in three challenging clinical contexts: withdrawing palliative chemotherapy, a request for assisted dying and the ethical challenges faced in a pandemic. The test of a clinical ethical model lies in its practical application in the clinical setting. The two clinical examples highlight the central role of the patient-doctor relationship, while the final example illustrates how relational ethics may foster trust and solidarity in the face of a pandemic.

Chapter 9 discusses ways in which the empathy-based ethical approach might be embedded in clinical practice, medical education and research. If, as has been argued, empathy is both important and desirable in clinical practice, the question arises as to how to enhance empathy between the doctor and patient. Initiatives to incorporate empathy into undergraduate medical education are reviewed, including a discussion on the role of the humanities and the impact of positive role models (Jeffrey 2019).

Patient-centred medicine has been defined as a form of practice seeking to focus medical attention on the individual patient's needs and concerns rather than those of the doctor (Bardes 2012). Patient-centred medicine involves adopting a phenomenological approach to practice where listening to and empathising with the patient's experience of their illness are paramount. Phenomenology involves empathy in its attempt to understand the patient's experience of their illness. Phenomenology inevitably includes the process of interpretation of the patient's narrative. The possibilities of incorporating a phenomenological approach into the doctor-patient relationship and into medical education are debated.

Research into empathy in medicine has mainly been restricted to quantitative studies, measuring doctors' and students' empathy based on self-reported questionnaires. The limitations of these studies are discussed as there is now a need for further qualitative research to explore the nuanced relational concept of empathy.

Chapter 10 looks to the future for empathy-based ethics (EBE) and its role in humanising medical care. Empathy is an experience which occurs between two people and is influenced by the context of their meeting. Humanising medicine can best be achieved by addressing the current biomedical-psychosocial imbalance and by adopting a relational approach of empathy-based ethics (EBE). Empathy-based ethics offers doctors and patients a more fulfilling relationship in which patients are truly involved in their care. Medical students, tomorrow's doctors, may also benefit by a greater emphasis on empathy-based ethics in their undergraduate curriculum.

REFERENCES

Bardes, C. L. (2012). Patient centred medicine. *New England Journal of Medicine, 366,* 782–783.

Batson, C. (2011). These things called empathy: Eight related but distinct phenomena. In J. Decety & W. Ickes (Eds.), *The social neuroscience of empathy* (pp. 6–15). Cambridge: MIT Press.

Bensing, J. (2000). Bridging the gap: The separate worlds of evidence-based medicine and patient-centred medicine. *Patient Education and Counseling, 39,* 17–25.

Berwick, D. M. (2016). Era 3 for medicine and health care. *Journal of the American Medical Association, 315*(13), 1329–1330.

Calderwood, C. (2016). *Realistic medicine: Chief Medical Officer's Annual Report 2014–15.* Edinburgh: Scottish Government.

Cambridge English Dictionary. (2020). *Cambridge English Dictionary.* Retrieved 6th May 2020, from https://dictionary.cambridge.org/dictionary/english/humanize?q=humanise.

Coplan, A., & Goldie, P. (Eds.). (2011). *Empathy: Philosophical and psychological perspectives*. Oxford: Oxford University Press.

Cummings, J., & Bennett, V. (2012). *Compassion in practice: Nursing, midwifery and care staff: Our vision and strategy*. London: NHS England.

Derksen, F., et al. (2013). Effectiveness of empathy in general practice: A systematic review. *British Journal General Practice, 63*, 76–84.

de Zulueta, P. (2013a). Compassion in 21st century medicine: Is it sustainable? *Clinical Ethics, 8*(4), 119–128.

de Zulueta, P. (2013b). Responding to the Francis Report: Some simple but radical suggestions. *Journal of Holistic Healthcare, 10*(1), 20–22.

Francis, R. (2013). *Report of the Mid Staffordshire NHS Foundation Trust public inquiry: Executive summary*. London: HMSO.

Halpern, J. (2001). *From detached concern to empathy: Humanizing medical practice*. Oxford: Oxford University Press.

Haque, O. S., & Waytz, A. (2012). Dehumanization in medicine: Causes, solutions and functions. *Perspectives on Psychological Science, 7*, 176–186.

Hojat, M., et al. (2009). The devil is in the third year: A longitudinal study of erosion of empathy in medical school. *Academic Medicine, 84*(9), 1182–1191.

Jeffrey, D. (2016). A meta-ethnography of interview-based qualitative research studies on medical students' views and experiences of empathy. *Medical Teacher, 38*(12), 1214–1220.

Jeffrey, D. I. (2019). *Exploring empathy with medical students*. London: Palgrave Macmillan.

Kearney, M. K., et al. (2009). Self-care of physicians caring for patients at the end of life "Being Connected … .A key to survival." *Journal of the American Medical Association, 301*, 1155–1164.

Macnaughton, J. (2009). The dangerous practice of empathy. *Lancet, 373*(9679), 1940–1941.

Mallia, P. (2013). *The nature of the doctor-patient relationship: Health care principles through the phenomenology of relationships with patients*. Dordrecht: Springer.

Marcum, J. A. (2008). *An introductory philosophy of medicine: Humanizing modern medicine*. Dortrecht: Springer.

Montgomery, K. (2006). *How doctors think: Clinical judgment and the practice of medicine*. Oxford: Oxford University Press.

Parliamentary Health Service Ombudsman. (2011). *Care and compassion?: Report of the Health Service Ombudsman on ten investigations into NHS care of older people*. London: HMSO.

Quince, T., et al. (2016). Undergraduate medical students' empathy: Current perspectives. *Advances in Medical Education and Practice, 7*, 443–455.

Simpson, P. D., & Morris, E. P. (2014). The implications of the Francis Report. *Obstetrics, Gynaecology & Reproductive Medicine, 24*, 186–188.

Sturzu, L., et al. (2019). Empathy and burnout—A cross-sectional study among mental healthcare providers in France. *Journal of Medicine and Life, 12*, 21–29.
Weatherall, D. (1994). The inhumanity of medicine. *BMJ, 309*, 1671.

CHAPTER 2

Humane Medicine

Abstract Humane medicine is a practice focusing on the whole patient and not simply their disease, reinstating the humanity of both patient and doctor. Dehumanisation is a denial of full human status to patients with resultant suffering. Dehumanisation may be manifest in subtle ways: a lack of personal care, an emphasis on technology, a lack of warmth and a focus on efficiency. Medicine's positivist view prioritises technical progress, evidence-based medicine, targets and efficiency, so risking a view of patients solely as objects of intellectual interest. Dehumanisation fails to see the patient as an individual, and patients become treated as a means to an end, losing their capacity to evoke empathy with a resultant psychological distancing by the doctor. The dominance of the biomedical approach has led to a form of medical professionalism described as detached concern. This model of detachment has contributed to dehumanisation of the patient.

Keywords Humane medicine · Dehumanisation · Detached concern · Biomedical approach

INTRODUCTION

This chapter examines what is meant by humane medicine and contrasts this by describing how patients may be dehumanised in subtle ways in everyday practice. After a brief case history illustrating such dehumanisation, the causes of such practice are discussed, highlighting how empathy-based ethics may lead to a more humane way of working.

HUMANE MEDICINE

Humanity, having a human nature, comprises a wide range of characteristics including emotional responsiveness, interpersonal warmth, cognitive openness and individual agency (Haslam 2006). Humane medicine acknowledges both patient and doctor as fellow human beings of equal moral worth. Most patients want a feeling of connection with their doctor; Anatole Broyard wrote of his doctor during his last illness:

> I just wish he would brood on my situation for perhaps five minutes, that he would give me his whole mind just once, be bonded with me for a brief space, survey my soul as well as my flesh, to get at my illness, for each man is ill in his own way. (Broyard 1992)

A director of the Patients Association identified five key factors that patients wanted from their doctors: eye contact, partnership, communication, time and access (Stone 2003). Each of these items relates to connection with the doctor in a special relationship rather than issues of technical competence. A doctor's competence is highly relevant to high standards of clinical practice, yet patients seem to take this for granted when discussing their relationship with doctors. A review of studies, investigating patients' views of a good doctor, found that patients rated 'fostering the relationship' a high priority (Deledda et al. 2013). Patients wanted to be recognised as individuals in a partnership with their doctor. This wish for a mutually respectful relationship was echoed in a qualitative study of patients with breast cancer (Wright et al. 2004). In this study, patients expressed a wish 'to be a human being, somebody who has an opinion' (Wright et al. 2004). Patients were more concerned with the doctor's enduring qualities rather than their communication skills, needing to feel safe in a caring relationship with a trusted expert. Given that most patients want a close relationship with their doctor, it is perhaps strange that some doctors perceive a need for detachment from them.

Humane medicine is a practice focusing on the whole patient and not simply their disease. It does not seek to reject the scientific aspects of care but in embracing psychological and social dimensions it reinstates the humanity of both patient and doctor (Marcum 2008). Authors have made a plea to make medicine relational by which they mean a practice which is partnership-orientated, responsive to the patient's needs and empathic (Davis-Floyd and Saint John 1998). Montgomery developed these arguments by acknowledging the benefits of biomedicine and proposing that clinical medicine be seen as an interpretative practice rather than as a pure science, involving a commitment to listen to the patient's story (Montgomery 2006). Listening to the patient's experience of their illness in an empathic relationship and interpreting their story are hallmarks of a phenomenological approach to practice.

Humane medicine acknowledges emotions and subjectivity as an integral part of practice, not a barrier to clinical decision-making. The patient is involved in decisions as a partner in a relationship of equals in a practice of empathic care. A humane doctor is both competent and empathic. Central to a humane approach, empathy enables a doctor to engage with the psychosocial features and meaning of a patient's illness: losses, anxiety and suffering (Toombs 1993). Respecting the patient as an autonomous person enables them to be involved in therapeutic decisions and contributes to the healing process. Humane medicine is based on an *ethos* of empathy which drives the *logos* (technical care). In contrast, the biomedical model focuses on the *logos* of medicine which determines an *ethos* of distancing (Marcum 2008).

INHUMANE MEDICINE

Twenty-five years ago, Weatherall argued that many of the ills of the medical profession reflected a lack of "whole person understanding" (Weatherall 1994). More recently, Spiro expressed concern that doctors who used to listen to patients now looked at a screen (Spiro 2009). Medicine's positivist view prioritises technical progress, evidence-based medicine, targets and efficiency, so risking a view of patients solely as objects of intellectual interest (Shapiro 2012). Mechanistic organisational healthcare systems may create a risk of dehumanisation, denying patient's dignity and alienating clinicians from patients (Borgstrom and Walter 2015; de Zulueta 2013a, b; Haslam 2015; Zigmond 2011).

Doctors complain that their ability to practice empathically is jeopardised by NHS bureaucracy, causing some patients to feel that their concerns are not addressed adequately (Greenhalgh et al. 2014; Howick and Rees 2017). Since empathy depends upon cognitive and emotional understanding of the patient, dehumanisation by treating others in a detached way can be equated with a lack of empathy (Haslam 2006). Treating patients in this mechanistic manner allows doctors to experience less moral concern for their actions and may seem to justify acts that would otherwise be considered harmful (Haslam 2006).

The question arises as to why people in caring professions cease to show care? (Haslam 2015). The contributory factors identified in the Francis Report included compassion fatigue, overwork, excess demand, lack of continuity and a failure to see the patient as a fellow human being (Francis 2013; Haslam 2015). Healthcare professionals may distance themselves from patients, avoiding emotions and focusing on biomedical facts, a process described as 'existential neglect' or 'detached concern' (Agledahl et al. 2011; de Zulueta 2013a; Halpern 2001). The blame culture prevalent in the NHS also contributes to a punitive climate, where a lack of tolerance and an inbuilt hierarchy may influence good people to act harmfully (de Zulueta 2013a).

Medical dehumanisation may be an unintended consequence rather than as a result of any malicious intent on the part of healthcare professionals. Unconscious, unintentional dehumanisation of patients can occur as a product of the organisational culture in hospitals and community settings (Haque and Waytz 2012).

HANNAH BUTLER'S STORY

Hannah Butler, a thirty-year-old teacher, makes an appointment to see Dr Jones, her GP. She is summoned to his office over the waiting room intercom. Flustered, she loses her way in the corridor, every door seems the same. Dr Jones opens the door of his consulting room,

"Good morning Mrs Butler, are you lost? Please come in".

Hannah Butler enters his office, sitting down she watches Dr Jones staring at the computer screen.

"Excuse me a moment, please, I am just checking your history and prescriptions. What is the problem today?"

"My asthma has been worse, I am not sleeping" replied Mrs Butler.

"I can see that you have not seen the practice nurse for an asthma check for over a year. Are you using both your brown steroid and the blue salbutamol inhalers?"

"No, I am so busy at work that I forget, I just use the blue one when I get wheezy".

"Let's measure your lung function today, could you please blow into this flowmeter for me?" asked Dr Jones.

As Mrs Butler reached for the flowmeter, Dr Jones noticed a recent burn on her wrist. He wondered whether to ask about the burn but decided it was better just to sort out her asthma, as the waiting room is full of patients and he is half an hour behind in his morning surgery.

"Thank you, the reading is a bit low so could you please restart the steroid inhaler twice a day and pop back to see sister Barnes in the asthma clinic next Thursday? Make an appointment on your way out at reception".

"Yes, that will be OK", replied Mrs Butler.

"I am sure you will feel better when your asthma is under control. Is there anything else?" asked Dr Jones.

"No. I suppose not...thank you, anyway". She replied.

This short scenario depicts a consultation dominated by the biomedical model of medicine, where the patient is not treated as a fellow human being but simply one who exhibits a problem of uncontrolled asthma. Psychosocial cues are ignored, revealing a lack of empathy and moral disengagement. The general practitioner shows a detached concern, addressing the disease, while ignoring the social context of the person in front of him. He controls the power in the consultation while failing to offer any personal continuity of care. He is ready to pass the patient on to another member of the healthcare team without offering her any choice in her management.

DEHUMANISATION

Dehumanisation is a strong term, yet in health care it is an everyday experience for some people, a denial of full human status to patients with resultant suffering (Haslam 2006). Treating people in a detached unfeeling way may deny their sense of dignity and displays a lack of empathy (Haque and Waytz 2012). Dehumanisation may be manifest in many subtle ways: a lack of personal care, an emphasis on technology, a lack of warmth and a focus on efficiency (Haslam 2006). It may be based on interventions performed on a passive patient whose autonomy is disregarded, a process described as "objectification" (Haslam 2006). "Objectification" may also reduce the doctor's sense of moral obligation to the patient. Nussbaum identified different ways of "objectification": treating patients as a means to an end, seeing them as lacking self-determination, stereotyping and believing that their feelings can be neglected (Nussbaum 1999). Dehumanisation sometimes may be used as a coping mechanism to deal with the personal distress of caring for dying patients (Haslam 2006).

EXAMPLES OF DEHUMANISATION

Denial of Individuality

Dehumanisation fails to see the patient as an individual, independent, distinguishable from others and capable of making choices (Kelman 1976). Patients become treated as a means to an end and so lose their capacity to evoke empathy (Opotow 1990). People's values express their distinctive humanity, but dehumanisation may be evident in 'in-group' and 'out-group' divisions where outsiders are perceived to lack shared humanity and their interests disregarded (Schwartz and Struch 1989).

Doctors whose individuality is denied may lead them to dehumanise patients (Haque and Waytz 2012). Doctors and medical students on a ward round may form an anonymous group surrounding the patient, making it difficult for anyone to challenge a consultant's patronising behaviour (Haque and Waytz 2012). Patients, dressed in scanty hospital gowns, identified by a wristband number, may appear anonymous rather than unique human beings requiring empathy (Haque and Waytz 2012). An inspirational doctor in elderly care had to start a campaign to ensure that doctors simply introduced themselves to patients: "Hello, my name is...." (Grainger 2013).

Detached Concern and the Mechanistic Biomedical Model

Mechanistic dehumanisation involves a denial of the humanity of the patient and a resultant psychological distancing by the doctor. This distancing is often accompanied by indifference, a lack of empathy and an abstract and intellectualised view (Haslam 2006). The notion that doctors should be emotionally detached from patients was endorsed by the famous physician Sir William Osler. "*This neutrality in witnessing human suffering gives him (the doctor) a special glimpse into the "inner life" of patients*" (Osler 1963). An opposing view was presented in 1927, in a seminal paper, Peabody claimed, "*One of the essential qualities of the clinician is interest in humanity, for the secret of the care of the patient is in caring for the patient*" (Peabody 1927).

Forty years ago, the problems of a reductionist positivist view in medical practice and its resultant disease-orientated, biomedical model were identified by Engel (Engel 1978). He commented on the doctor's failure to see the patient as a person and proposed changing the prevailing medical culture to a patient-orientated biopsychosocial model of care. However, the dominance of the biomedical model in medicine persists and there is now an urgent need to redress the balance between scientific and psychosocial care (de Zulueta 2013a).

Medical problem solving sometimes does entail focusing on a physical part of the patient and disregarding a person's inner mental life, e.g. during surgery. However, there is a risk that in a routine physical examination of the patient, a doctor may treat the patient like an object rather than a unique individual (Haque and Waytz 2012). Doctors sometimes have to cause some harms to patients which may be justified by the resulting benefit. For example, a woman may accept the need for mutilating surgery or toxic chemotherapy in order to survive a breast cancer. Doctors seeking to minimise their guilt of inflicting pain may dehumanise the patient, since by viewing patients as less capable of emotional feelings, they may feel less guilty (Haque and Waytz 2012).

The association between the biomedical approach and distancing from patients was a finding in a qualitative study of oncologists' approaches to end of life care (Jackson et al. 2008). The authors found that doctors who combined both biomedical and psychosocial aspects of care described having a connected relationship with the patient (Jackson et al. 2008). However, doctors who described primarily a biomedical role reported a more distant relationship with the patient (Jackson et al. 2008). Montgomery concluded that the biomedical emphasis caused an unnecessary impersonal form of clinical practice, dissatisfied patients and disheartened doctors (Montgomery 2006).

Patient-Doctor Dissimilarity

Labelling the patient as an illness, a 'diabetic' rather than as a unique individual who has diabetes, dehumanises because it fosters a view of the patient as a disease and creates a difference between the patient and the healthy doctor (Haque and Waytz 2012). Power differences between the patient and doctor may be a result of the patient's vulnerability and sense of loss of control. The contrasting authority of the doctor may lead the patient to adopt a passive role (Marcum 2008).

Illnesses may alter the patient's appearance, behaviour and basic functioning all factors contributing to further disparity from the doctor and the potential for dehumanisation. People are more likely to dehumanise those who appear different from them (Haque and Waytz 2012).

Medical Undergraduate Education

There is a perception in medical education research that medical students' empathy declines during their undergraduate training (Batt-Rawden et al. 2013; Hojat et al. 2009; Neumann et al. 2011; Pedersen 2009). This view is challenged by recent qualitative research (Jeffrey 2018; Quince et al. 2016). Students' stories show that the biomedical model of medical care persists in their undergraduate curriculum, with a resultant neglect of psychosocial aspects of care (Epstein 2014; Jeffrey 2016, 2018; Montgomery 2006). The over-riding commitment to scientific academic medicine can lead to the development of a 'biomedical gaze' (Jeffrey 2019; Pedersen 2010). This scientific stance reflects the dominant discourse, where medicine is concerned largely with giving objective advice rather than connecting with the patient. The suppression of empathy risks becoming seen as a desirable skill for a physician (Hardy 2017). Such physicians, who embody a detached scientific attitude, can be role models for students, who, in turn, lose empathy with patients (Hardy 2017). It seems, therefore, that adopting the scientific biomedical model exclusively can contribute to detachment and a lack of empathy.

In a recent study, students described how the patient's experience seemed to be added on at the end of lectures simply as a token, if it was addressed at all. They also related that during ward rounds clinicians appeared to be concerned with symptoms and signs rather than the psychological needs of patients (Jeffrey 2018). Students realised that they often lost sight of the uniqueness of the individual patient in a clinical environment focused on efficiency (Head et al. 2012; Sood and Moore 2019; Wear and Zarconi 2008).

Students commented that evidence-based guidelines were another mechanism for emphasising scientific aspects of medicine rather than listening to the patient's experience (Eikeland et al. 2014; Michalec 2011). There seems to be a risk that the strong emphasis on scientific facts might alienate students from their own feelings, undermining opportunities for reflection (Eikeland et al. 2014). However, authors have argued that evidence-based medicine (EBM) must be integrated with clinical experience and humane care in the practice of clinical judgement (Bensing 2000; Montgomery 2006).

In summary, the biomedical emphasis in the curriculum seemed to have two main effects on the students: it caused them distress by neglecting psychosocial aspects of the patient's suffering and distanced them from patients who were sometimes seen as objects of intellectual interest (Jeffrey 2019).

Conclusion

The dominance of biomedical approach in medical practice and education has led to a form of medical professionalism described as detached concern (Halpern 2001). This model of detachment has contributed to dehumanisation of the patient. Patients want emotional connection in their relationship with doctors. At the heart of this connection is the experience of empathy. In the next chapter, the complex nature of empathy and its core role in relational ethics are explored.

References

Agledahl, K. M., et al. (2011). Courteous but not curious: How doctors' politeness masks their existential neglect. A qualitative study of video-recorded patient consultations. *Journal of Medical Ethics, 37*(11), 650–654.

Batt-Rawden, S., et al. (2013). Teaching empathy to medical students: An updated, systematic review. *Academic Medicine, 88*(8), 1171–1177.

Bensing, J. (2000). Bridging the gap: The separate worlds of evidence-based medicine and patient-centred medicine. *Patient Education and Counseling, 39*, 17–25.

Borgstrom, E., & Walter, T. (2015). Choice and compassion at the end of life: A critical analysis of recent English policy discourse. *Social Science and Medicine, 136*, 99–105.

Broyard, A. (1992). *Intoxicated by my illness: And other writings on life and death*. New York: Fawcett Columbine.

Davis-Floyd, R., & Saint John, G. (1998). *From doctor to healer: The transformative journey*. London: Rutgers University Press.

Deledda, G., et al. (2013). How patients want their doctors to communicate. A literature review on primary care patients' perspective. *Patient Education and Counseling, 90,* 297–306.

de Zulueta, P. (2013a). Compassion in 21st century medicine: Is it sustainable? *Clinical Ethics, 8*(4), 119–128.

de Zulueta, P. (2013b). Responding to the Francis Report: Some simple but radical suggestions. *Journal of Holistic Healthcare, 10*(1), 20–22.

Eikeland, H. L., et al. (2014). The physician's role and empathy—A qualitative study of third year medical students. *BMC Medical Education, 14,* 165–173.

Engel, G. L. (1978). The biopsychosocial model and the education of health professionals. *Annals of the New York Academy of Sciences, 310*(1), 169–181.

Epstein, R. M. (2014). Realizing Engel's biopsychosocial vision: Resilience, compassion, and quality of care. *The International Journal of Psychiatry in Medicine, 47*(4), 275–287.

Francis, R. (2013). *Report of the Mid Staffordshire NHS Foundation Trust public inquiry: Executive summary*. London: HMSO.

Grainger, K. (2013). *Hello my name is*. Retrieved 23rd September 2020, from https://www.hellomynameis.org.uk/.

Greenhalgh, T., et al. (2014). Evidence based medicine: A movement in crisis? *BMJ, 348,* g3725.

Halpern, J. (2001). *From detached concern to empathy: Humanizing medical practice*. Oxford: Oxford University Press.

Haque, O. S., & Waytz, A. (2012). Dehumanization in medicine: Causes, solutions and functions. *Perspectives on Psychological Science, 7,* 176–186.

Hardy, C. (2017). Empathizing with patients: The role of interaction and narratives in providing better patient care. *Medicine, Healthcare and Philosophy, 20,* 237–248.

Haslam, D. (2015). More than kindness. *Journal of Compassionate Health Care, 2*(1), 6–9.

Haslam, N. (2006). Dehumanization: An integrative review. *Personality and Social Psychology Review, 10,* 252–264.

Head, B. A., et al. (2012). "I will never forget": What we learned from medical student reflections on a palliative care experience. *Journal of Palliative Medicine, 15*(5), 535–541.

Hojat, M., et al. (2009). The devil is in the third year: A longitudinal study of erosion of empathy in medical school. *Academic Medicine, 84*(9), 1182–1191.

Howick, J., & Rees, S. (2017). Overthrowing barriers to empathy in healthcare: Empathy in the age of the internet. *Journal of the Royal Society of Medicine, 110*, 352–357.

Jackson, V., et al. (2008). A qualitative study of oncologists' approaches to end-of-life care. *Journal of Palliative Medicine, 11*(6), 893–906.

Jeffrey, D. (2016). A meta-ethnography of interview-based qualitative research studies on medical students' views and experiences of empathy. *Medical Teacher, 38*(12), 1214–1220.

Jeffrey, D. (2018). *Exploring empathy with medical students: A qualitative longitudinal phenomenological study* (PhD thesis). University of Edinburgh.

Jeffrey, D. I. (2019). *Exploring empathy with medical students*. London: Palgrave Macmillan.

Kelman, H. C. (1976). Violence without restraint: Reflections on the dehumanization of victims and victimizers. In G. M. Kren & L. Rappoport (Eds.), *Varieties of psychohistory*. New York: Springer.

Marcum, J. A. (2008). *An introductory philosophy of medicine: Humanizing modern medicine*. Dortrecht: Springer.

Michalec, B. (2011). Learning to cure, but learning to care? *Advances in Health Sciences Education, 16*(1), 109–130.

Montgomery, K. (2006). *How doctors think: Clinical judgment and the practice of medicine*. Oxford: Oxford University Press.

Neumann, M., et al. (2011). Empathy decline and its reasons: A systematic review of studies with medical students and residents. *Academic Medicine, 86*(8), 996–1009.

Nussbaum, M. C. (1999). *Sex and social justice*. Oxford: Oxford University Press.

Opotow, S. (1990). Moral exclusion and injustice: An introduction. *Journal of Social Issues, 46*, 1–20.

Osler, W. (1963). *Aequanimitas*. New York: Nortop.

Peabody, F. (1927). The care of the patient. *Journal of the American Medical Association, 88*, 876–882.

Pedersen, R. (2009). Empirical research on empathy in medicine—A critical review. *Patient Education and Counseling, 76*(3), 307–322.

Pedersen, R. (2010). Empathy development in medical education—A critical review. *Medical Teacher, 32*(7), 593–600.

Quince, T., et al. (2016). Undergraduate medical students' empathy: Current perspectives. *Advances in Medical Education and Practice, 7*, 443–455.

Schwartz, S. H., & Struch, N. (1989). Values, stereotypes, and intergroup antagonism. In D. Bar-Tal, C. F. Grauman, A. W. Kruglanski, & W. Stroebe (Eds.), *Stereotypes and prejudice: Changing conceptions*. New York: Springer-Verlag.

Shapiro, J. (2012). The paradox of teaching empathy in medical students. In J. Decety (Ed.), *Empathy: From bench to bedside*. Cambridge: MIT Press.

Sood, M., & Moore, J. (2019, March). Empathy, emotional attachment, and the end. *British Journal of General Practice, 69,* 132.

Spiro, H. (2009). Commentary: The practice of empathy. *Academic Medicine, 84*(9), 1177–1179.

Stone, M. (2003). What patients want from their doctors. *BMJ, 326,* 1294.

Toombs, S. K. (1993). *The meaning of Illness: A phenomenological account of the different perspectives of physician and patient.* Dordrecht, The Netherlands: Kluwer.

Wear, D., & Zarconi, J. (2008). Can compassion be taught? Let's ask our students. *Journal of General Internal Medicine, 23*(7), 948–953.

Weatherall, D. (1994). The inhumanity of medicine. *BMJ, 309,* 1671.

Wright, E. B., et al. (2004). Doctors communication of trust, care and respect in breast cancer: A qualitative study. *BMJ, 328,* 864.

Zigmond, D. (2011). Five executive follies: How commodification imperils compassion in person healthcare. *Journal Holistic Healthcare, 9,* 7–10.

CHAPTER 3

Empathy: A Relational Experience

Abstract The focus in this book is on empathy between a doctor and patient, but the empathy-based ethical approach applies to the relationship between a patient and any healthcare professional. The history of the concept of empathy is briefly reviewed. Broad models of empathy describe four overlapping dimensions: affective, cognitive, behavioural and moral. Medicine's positivist philosophy fosters a cognitive form of empathy or 'detached concern' as the appropriate mode of medical professionalism, but empathy is better regarded as a dynamic relational construct, dependent upon context. Caring involves some degree of identification with another person as a human being with needs and deserving respect; this is part of the moral force of empathy.

Keywords Relational empathy · Detached concern · Evolution of empathy

INTRODUCTION

Empathy is a complex dynamic concept which has been defined in the literature in many ways. If doctors are to respond to calls to provide more compassionate care, there is a need for clarity. The conceptualisation of empathy has evolved differently in medicine, nursing, philosophy,

21

D. I. Jeffrey, *Empathy-Based Ethics*,
https://doi.org/10.1007/978-3-030-64804-6_3

psychology and counselling. In this book, the focus is on empathy between a doctor and patient, but the ethical approach applies to the relationship between a patient and any healthcare professional.

THE EVOLUTION OF EMPATHY

Theodor Lipps (1851–1914) adopted the term *Einfühlung* (feeling into) from aesthetics, to explain how people became aware of each other's mental states, with an emphasis on emotional (affective) aspects of empathy (Lipps 1903). *Einfühlung*, according to Lipps, was a process of imitation, or inner resonance, with the other person, an "emotional contagion" (Lipps 1903). In 1909, Edward Tichner (1867–1927) used the Greek word *empatheia* to translate *Einfühlung* and was first to introduce the term 'empathy' (Tichner 1909).

Initially, empathy was seen as a concept involving emotions, but early in the twentieth century, in phenomenological philosophy, it became associated with understanding, *"verstehen"*. Phenomenologists such as Husserl (1859–1938), Stein (1891–1942) and Scheler (1874–1928) were concerned with the vexed question of intersubjectivity, the problem of other minds (Coplan and Goldie 2011). For Husserl, empathy was a unique mode of consciousness through which others' thoughts, emotions and desires were directly experienced, enabling others to be viewed as 'minded' (Husserl 1989; Stein 1989). He saw empathy as an understanding of the meaning of the other person's shared humanity (Hooker 2015).

Stein further developed the concept of empathy by postulating that it enabled us not only to understand others, but also to understand ourselves as others experience us, adding a relational dimension to empathy (Stein 1989). Stein described empathy as 'happening' to us, somewhat like falling in love, i.e. a process that could not be forced (Davis 1990). She outlined a process of empathy in three stages: seeing the world from the other person's point of view, a sudden 'crossing over' involving an emotional shift with deep understanding and finally, regaining a self-other boundary (Davis 1990; Stein 1989).

From a clinical perspective, Carl Rogers (1899–1959), a founder of humanistic psychology, placed empathy at the heart of his patient-centred psychotherapy. Rogers claimed that empathy occurred when the therapist viewed patients with an "unconditional positive regard" (Rogers 1959). He proposed that when we empathise, we enter the world of the other and become at home in it, stressing the relational nature of empathy and pointing out the risk of over-identifying with the patient (Rogers 1961). He argued that an empathetic encounter depended upon maintaining a 'self-other' distinction (Rogers 1961).

Martin Buber (1878–1965) was also influential in promoting the affective elements of empathy in his description of an 'I/Thou relationship', rather than the objective 'I/It' in a process he called "dialogue" (Buber 2004). In the process of "dialogue", one person becomes closely connected to the other in a moment of shared meaning (Buber 1961).

Schutz (1899–1959) expanded the concept of empathy by focusing attention on the shared context where two subjects interact and affect each other in a face-to-face encounter, creating a 'we-relationship' (Schutz 1967).

These early, relational, affective views of empathy may be contrasted with the way in which empathy is now generally viewed in a medical context.

Medical Empathy

Empathy has largely been accepted in medical literature as an innate, personal attribute, subject to measurement (Baron-Cohen 2011; Hojat 2016; Hojat et al. 2009). Less commonly, it has been described as a dynamic reciprocal process (Irving and Dickson 2004). Broad models of empathy describe four dimensions: affective, cognitive, behavioural and moral (Morse et al. 1992). However, in practice, these four dimensions interact and overlap in differing clinical situations.

Cognitive

In contrast to the early phenomenological approaches to empathy where the emotional, relational and contextual nature of empathy is stressed, present medical practice has adopted a cognitive view of empathy which excludes emotional aspects.

> Empathy is a predominantly cognitive (rather than emotional) attribute that involves an understanding (rather than feeling) of experiences, concerns and perspectives of the patient, combined with a capacity to communicate this understanding. An intention to help by preventing and

alleviating pain and suffering is an additional feature of empathy in the context of patient care. (Hojat et al. 2009, p. 1183)

Hojat claims that taking a purely cognitive view enables empathy to be researched and measured scientifically (Hojat 2016).

we cannot scientifically study empathy in patient care unless an agreement exists concerning its definition and unless a psychometrically sound instrument is available to measure the defined concept. (Hojat 2016, p. 72)

Cognitive empathy is the ability to identify and understand another person's feelings and perspective from an objective stance, sometimes described as a capacity "to be in the other's shoes" (Shapiro 2008). In a medical context, cognitive empathy has been also described as "detached concern", or the ability of one individual to understand the experiences of another without evoking a personal emotional response (Neumann et al. 2012). Medicine's positivist philosophy, prioritising technical progress, fosters a cognitive form of empathy or 'detached concern' as the appropriate mode of medical professionalism (Halpern 2001; Shapiro et al. 2015).

Affective

It seems natural for doctors to adopt a form of empathy which included emotions, since much of medicine is concerned with the relief of suffering (Jeffrey 2016). Affective empathy is the ability to subjectively experience and share in another's psychological state or feelings (Morse et al. 1992). Sharing the emotion leads to empathic concern which precedes and contributes to helping behaviour (Eisenberg 2000).

In affective matching, the doctor experiences the same type of emotion as the patient. This matching is not simply an "emotional contagion" which is an involuntary spread of feelings without conscious awareness of their origin. Affective matching involves cognitive evaluation and imagination; we "catch" an emotion and experience it as our own (Coplan and Goldie 2011). Our emotional lives are linked to our actions, so there cannot be a rigid distinction between action and attitude. Empathy can be viewed as a form of perception where people can literally feel the emotional states of others as their own (Wisnewski 2015). Empathy can be thought of as a kind of human experience (Wisnewski 2015). Despite a shift in recent years towards an interest in the emotions of the patient, some authors still express reservations about emotional empathy (Betzler 2018).

Behavioural Empathy

Empathic concern motivates altruistic behaviour, in connecting with others we are motivated to act in response to the other's needs (Batson et al. 2009). Irving's three-dimensional model of empathy proposes that the doctor has to understand the patient's world (cognitive), feel with the patient (affective) and communicate this understanding with the patient (behavioural) (Irving and Dickson 2004).

Moral Empathy

In the 1980s, second-wave feminist 'care ethics' added a moral dimension to empathy, maintaining that in attempting to understand a situation from another person's point of view, moral behaviour required both reason and emotion (Gilligan 1982; Noddings 1984; Slote 2007). From this perspective, to care for another involved 'feeling with' the other person, which resonates with the concept of *Einfühlung* and a relational view of empathy (Lipps 1903; Stein 1989). Morse identifies a moral component as a fourth dimension of empathy: an internal motivation of concern for the other and a desire to act to relieve their suffering by caring (Morse et al. 1992). Empathy connects people in a way that promotes their well-being and increases the doctor's motivation for altruism (Batson 1991; Maxwell 2008).

From a care ethics perspective, the practice of caring is integral to moral life. Noddings thought that empathy was essential for developing an understanding of others and enabling clinical decision-making (Noddings 1984). For Noddings, care closely relates to empathy since caring depends upon attending to the specific needs of particular patients and attempting to understand the situation from their point of view (Noddings 1984). Hilfiker argues that a fundamental goal of teaching ethics in medicine should be to foster a sense of empathy (Hilfiker 2001).

Relational Views of Empathy

What is empathy? Its definition is a source of controversy amongst philosophers, psychologists and clinicians (van Dijke et al. 2019). In the medical literature, empathy is viewed largely as a personal cognitive attribute, but is better regarded as a dynamic relational construct, dependent upon context. There has been an attempt to move from detached concern towards incorporating emotional aspects of empathy in recent years, in response to patients' wishes for emotionally warm interactions with doctors (Underman and Hirshfield 2016; Vinson and Underman 2020).

Broad definitions of empathy propose that the doctor should try to understand the patient's world, share their feelings and communicate this understanding to them (Derksen et al. 2013; Irving and Dickson 2004). Some authors have extended the broad view of empathy to include taking action to help the patient (Decety 2011). Coplan summarises by defining empathy, "Empathy is a complex imaginative process in which an observer simulates another person's situated psychological state (both cognitive and affective) while maintaining a clear self-other differentiation" (Coplan and Goldie 2011).

However, these definitions do not indicate the extent of emotional sharing between the doctor and the patient. It is not clear if a doctor shares the feelings of a patient or merely identifies them. Halpern argues that a crucial part of empathy is to recognise what it feels like to experience emotions rather than merely labelling them (Halpern 2003).

Being human means being in caring relationships with other people (van Dijke et al. 2019). Empathy offers an opportunity to transcend ourselves and to connect with the inner world, thoughts and feelings of others.

Conclusion

This book argues for a broad relational concept of empathy, accounting for both the doctor and the patient, in the context of their meeting. Empathy, as a relational concept, comprises the following features (Jeffrey 2016):

- Connection: involving emotional sharing with the patient.
- Clinical curiosity: gaining insight into the patient's concerns, feelings and distress.
- Concern: for the patient which gives the patient a sense that they matter.
- An other-orientated perspective: the doctor tries to imagine what it is like to be the patient and to see the world from the patient's perspective.
- Self-other differentiation: this respects the patient as an individual with dignity.
- Reciprocity: a two-way relationship with the other.
- Reflection: taking a broader view.
- Care: acting on the understanding gained to help the patient.
- Humility: acknowledging the limits of one's empathy.

Appropriate support can help to give healthcare professionals the courage to enter the interpersonal world and practice empathic skills. Empathy is not something that just happens to us, it is a choice to make to pay attention to extend ourselves. It can be thought of as a human experience. It requires an effort (Jamison 2014).

A relational model of empathy focuses on developing skills, attitudes and moral concern rather than just encouraging students and doctors to be more compassionate (Halpern 2001). By accepting rather than resisting their own emotions, doctors can stay involved in care without despair (Halpern 2001). Caring involves some degree of identification with another person as a human being with needs and deserving respect; this is part of the moral force of empathy (Darley and Batson 1973). Empathy is related to sympathy, compassion, generosity, kindness and humility, relational virtues that are examined in the next chapter.

REFERENCES

Baron-Cohen, S. (2011). *Zero degrees of empathy*. London: Allen Lane.
Batson, C. D. (1991). *The altruism question: Toward a social-psychological answer*. Hillsdale, NJ: Lawrence Erlbaum Associates.
Batson, C. D., et al. (2009). Empathy and altruism. In C. Snyder & S. Lopez (Eds.), *Oxford handbook of positive psychology* (pp. 417–427). Oxford: Oxford University Press.

Betzler, R. J. (2018). How to clarify the aims of empathy in medicine. *Medicine, Health Care and Philosophy, 21,* 569–582.

Buber, M. (1961). *Between man and man.* London: Collins.

Buber, M. (2004). *I and thou.* London: Continuum.

Coplan, A., & Goldie, P. (Eds.). (2011). *Empathy: Philosophical and psychological perspectives.* Oxford: Oxford University Press.

Darley, J. M., & Batson, C. D. (1973). "From Jerusalem to Jericho": A study of situational and dispositional variables in helping behavior. *Journal of Personality and Social Psychology, 27*(1), 100.

Davis, C. M. (1990). What is empathy, and can empathy be taught? *Physical Therapy, 70*(11), 707–711.

Decety, J. (2011). *Empathy: From bench to bedside.* Cambridge: MIT Press.

Derksen, F., et al. (2013). Effectiveness of empathy in general practice: A systematic review. *British Journal General Practice, 63,* 76–84.

Eisenberg, N. (2000). Emotion, regulation, and moral development. *Annual Review of Psychology, 51*(1), 665–697.

Gilligan, C. (1982). *In a different voice: Psychological theory and women' development.* Cambridge: Harvard University Press.

Halpern, J. (2001). *From detached concern to empathy: Humanizing medical practice.* Oxford: Oxford University Press.

Halpern, J. (2003). What is clinical empathy? *Journal of General Internal Medicine, 18*(8), 670–674.

Hilfiker, D. (2001). From the victim's point of view. *Journal of Medical Humanities, 22*(4), 255–263.

Hojat, M. (2016). *Empathy in health profession education and primary care.* New York: Springer.

Hojat, M., et al. (2009). The devil is in the third year: A longitudinal study of erosion of empathy in medical school. *Academic Medicine, 84*(9), 1182–1191.

Hooker, C. (2015). Understanding empathy: Why phenomenology and hermeneutics can help medical education and practice. *Medicine, Health Care and Philosophy, 18*(4), 541–552.

Husserl, E. (1989). *Ideas pertaining to a pure phenomenology and to a phenomenological philosophy.* Second Book Studies in the Phenomenology of constitution. Dordrecht: Kluwer Academic Publishers.

Irving, P., & Dickson, D. (2004). Empathy: Towards a conceptual framework for health professionals. *International Journal of Health Care Quality Assurance, 17*(4), 212–220.

Jamison, L. (2014). *The empathy exams.* London: Granta.

Jeffrey, D. (2016). Clarifying empathy: The first step to more humane clinical care. *British Journal of General Practice, 66,* 101–102.

Lipps, T. (1903). *Asthetik.* Leipzig, Germany: Leopold Voss Verlag.

Maxwell, B. (2008). *Professional ethics education: Studies in compassionate empathy*. New York: Springer.

Morse, J. M., et al. (1992). Exploring empathy: A conceptual fit for nursing practice? *the Journal of Nursing Scholarship, 24*(4), 273–280.

Neumann, M., et al. (2012). Physician empathy: Definition, outcome-relevance and its measurement in patient care and medical education. *GMS Zeitschrift fur medizinische Ausbildung, 29*(1), 1–21.

Noddings, N. (1984). *Caring: A feminine approach to ethics and moral education*. Berkeley: University of California Press.

Rogers, C. R. (1959). A theory of therapy, personality and interpersonal relationships as developed in the client-centered framework. In S. E. Koch (Ed.), *Psychology: A study of science: Formulations of the person and the social context* (Vol. 3). New York: McGraw-Hill.

Rogers, C. R. (1961). *On becoming a person*. London: Constable.

Schutz, A. (1967). *The phenomenology of the social world*. Evanston, IL: Northwestern University Press.

Shapiro, J. (2008). Walking a mile in their patients' shoes: Empathy and othering in medical students' education. *Philosophy, Ethics, and Humanities in Medicine, 3*, 10–21.

Shapiro, J., et al. (2015). Medical professionalism: What the study of literature can contribute to the conversation. *Philosophy, Ethics, and Humanities in Medicine, 10*(1), 1.

Slote, M. (2007). *The ethics of care and empathy*. London: Routledge.

Stein, E. (1989). *On the problem of empathy (The collected works of Edith Stein Vol 3)*. Washington, DC: ICS Publishers.

Tichner, E. (1909). *Lectures on the experimental psychology of the thought processes*. New York: Macmillan.

Underman, K., & Hirshfield, L. E. (2016). Detached concern?: Emotional socialization in twenty-first century medical education. *Social Science and Medicine, 160*, 94–101.

van Dijke, J., et al. (2019). Care ethics: An ethics of empathy? *Nursing Ethics, 26*, 1282–1291.

Vinson, A. H., & Underman, K. (2020). Clinical empathy as emotional labor in medical work. *Social Science & Medicine, 251*, 112904.

Wisnewski, J. J. (2015). Perceiving sympathetically: Moral perception, embodiment, and medical ethics. *Journal of Medical Humanities, 36*(4), 309–319.

CHAPTER 4

Relational Virtues and Empathy

Abstract The close relationship between empathy, compassion, sympathy, kindness, generosity and humility is explored. Compassion is a deep awareness of the suffering of oneself and of other living beings coupled by the wish to relieve it. The differences between empathy and compassion are discussed and an argument put forward for retaining empathy as the fundamental core of a clinical ethical approach. Sympathy is a broad term, signifying a general fellow feeling which differs from empathy in taking a "self-orientated" perspective. Kindness is a virtue linked to compassion, generosity, benevolence, altruism and empathy. Generosity is the virtue of giving good things to others freely. Humility requires us to value our own worth appropriately while accepting our helplessness. Humility, like empathy and kindness, is a construct which connects doctors and patients.

Keywords Empathy · Compassion · Sympathy · Kindness · Humility · Generosity

© The Author(s), under exclusive license to Springer Nature
Switzerland AG 2020
D. I. Jeffrey, *Empathy-Based Ethics*,
https://doi.org/10.1007/978-3-030-64804-6_4

INTRODUCTION

Human social relationships and subjective emotions may be difficult to define. Empathy and compassion are often confused with each other and with a number of other processes involving sharing in another person's feelings, especially of distress or suffering (de Zulueta 2015; Maxwell 2008). This chapter examines the relationship between empathy and compassion—terms that are defined and conceptualised in many different ways in the literature and in everyday speech (Gladkova 2010). The close link between them is reflected in Maxwell's term "compassionate empathy", an attempt to clarify by adopting the broadest term (Maxwell 2008). This conceptual confusion has practical implications for clinical practice, research and medical education. Empathy also shares characteristics of other relational virtues such as sympathy, kindness, generosity and humility.

COMPASSION

Compassion, a word derived from the Latin meaning 'to suffer with', has like empathy varied and confusing definitions in the literature. Gilbert describes compassion as a deep awareness of the suffering of oneself and of other living beings coupled by the wish to relieve it (Gilbert 2009). Compassion has religious overtones particularly in Christian and Buddhist philosophy. Compassion like sympathy is evoked when something bad happens to another person, but compassion is generated by more serious states, implying a desire to help, yet not necessarily resulting in a helping action (Gladkova 2010).

Compassion, like empathy, highlights engagement and a wish to relieve suffering, reflecting our need for social relationships (Batson 2011). In its drive to alleviate suffering, compassion shares elements with altruism. However, one can feel compassionate concern for another without making any attempt to understand their feelings and point of view.

EMPATHY AND COMPASSION: THE DIFFERENCES

For some authors, empathy is a part compassion, while others feel compassion is a result of empathy (Charlton 2016; de Zulueta 2013). Others view compassion has having cognitive components which make its differentiation from empathy unclear (Batson 2011). Smajdor conflates compassion with emotional empathy, linking it with distress and burnout (Smajdor et al. 2011). Authors taking a purely cognitive view of empathy see compassion as the emotional component of the encounter between doctor and patient (Warmington 2012).

The current use of the term empathy in health care is at risk of being equated with empathy in the limited cognitive sense (Kohut 1984; Wispé 1986). This approach reduces the affective component of empathy, whereas the word compassion puts the emotional element at its core. However, compassion crucially lacks cognitive elements integral to empathy (Halpern 2001). Motivation in compassion may be misguided, unlike empathy, which requires understanding of the other's view and so forms a part of *phronesis* or practical wisdom. Some authors argue that the motivation to help in compassion creates a distinction from empathy, but altruism is integral to relational empathy (de Zulueta 2013).

Contemporary social psychology literature admits a distinction between empathy, sympathy and compassion, but then treats them as variations of the same broad affective phenomena, referred to as empathy (Batson et al. 1995). Maxwell summarises this confusing situation "When it comes to 'empathy' the waters of terminological confusion run deep indeed" (Maxwell 2008). Empathy, as a relational construct is the preferable term to 'sympathy' or 'compassion' in clinical care since it is dynamic, accounts for affective and cognitive domains, involves action and has a central moral role (Jeffrey 2016a).

Empathy does include elements of sympathy and compassion but it also carries pertinent connotations that both sympathy and compassion lack (Maxwell 2008). It appears that affective elements of empathy, in particular, overlap with compassion and sympathy. Empathy clearly involves imaginative involvement, and although it is possible for both sympathy and compassion to be mediated by imaginative involvement, these terms typically refer to reactive and unreflective responses whose features require no great psychological acumen to appreciate. Empathy seems to suggest a response to situations whose features are more subtle, imperceptible and complex which require both affective and cognitive skills to perceive, share and understand. Empathy is a skilled response while sympathy and compassion are reactive responses which is why developing the skill of empathy is a more realistic educational goal, whereas teaching compassion seems counterintuitive (Maxwell 2008). For Maxwell, empathy involves capacities of moral sensitivity, both opening oneself to the other's subjective experience and getting judgements about the other's subjective experience right, empathic accuracy (Maxwell 2008). Maxwell's 'compassionate empathy' does not resolve this conceptual confusion. A more practical solution is to develop a *relational* conceptualisation of empathy, of particular relevance in medicine, where empathy encompasses a sense of feeling of distress in solidarity with a suffering person (Jeffrey 2016a; Maxwell 2008).

Empathy is the preferred term because empathy, more than sympathy and compassion, connotes not just reactive distress at another's suffering but considered and justified 'rational distress' (Maxwell 2008). The doctor is able to resonate with the patient's emotions yet remain aware of what is distinct in the patient's experience. Empathy is a form of engagement that seeks both cognitively and affectively to make sense of another's experience while preserving and respecting a self-other boundary. In contrast, compassion does not necessarily involve cognitive understanding of the others' views. Furthermore, the empirical nature of compassion is not well understood, it involves the presence of suffering and a desire to relieve it in a dynamic relationship which may change over time. There is an inherent tension in linking the intangible nature of compassion to concrete institutional initiatives mandating compassion as a right (Francis 2013).

SYMPATHY

Sympathy is the broadest of these terms, signifying a general fellow feeling, no matter of what kind. It is an emotion caused by the realisation that something bad has happened to another person, from mild discomfort to serious suffering (Gladkova 2010). In defining empathy, some authors contrast the concept with sympathy, which has been defined as experiencing another's emotions, as opposed to imagining those emotions (Stepien and Baernstein 2006). It has also been described as concern for the welfare of others (Jean Decety et al. 2010). Some authors feel sympathy is a wholly distinct concept from empathy, while others maintain that sympathy overlaps with the emotional component of empathy (Halpern 2001; Hojat et al. 2001; Mercer and Reynolds 2002). Sympathy may slide into a feeling of pity, or feeling sorry for the other person (Smajdor et al. 2011).

Sympathy differs crucially from empathy in taking a "self-orientated" perspective which may arise from an egoistic motivation to help the other person in order to relieve one's own distress. In taking such a self-orientated perspective, the doctor risks being personally distressed or even overwhelmed (Hojat et al. 2009).

KINDNESS

Kindness is an elusive concept which is easy to recognise but difficult to define. Kindness is a virtue linked to compassion, generosity, benevolence, altruism and empathy (Haskins and Thomas 2018). It is derived from kinship or concern for fellow human beings and acts as a connection between the self and the other (Jeffrey 2016b). Ballatt argues that kindness is no soft option but inspires people to build relationships with patients and to treat them well (Ballatt and Campling 2011). Kindness can have negative associations with patronising behaviour, pity or paternalism. It may also be regarded with suspicion as either a self-serving behaviour or a form of weakness as it often involves exposing our own vulnerability (Jeffrey 2016b).

Unkindness is often hard to challenge in a medical hierarchy where it can extend to bullying and harassment. Unkindness to patients is often subtle, by using distancing tactics such as appearing busy and disregarding a patient's anxieties; doctors can leave patients feeling isolated and dehumanised. It is paradoxical that we have developed sophisticated methods of communication but at a personal level these seem to have isolated us from others. We find it difficult to find another human being to speak face to face, to touch, to listen, to share our thoughts and to connect. Independence and self-reliance are now our ethical aspirations. Philips et al. ask "What is it about our times that makes kindness seem so dangerous?" (Philips and Taylor 2009).

We have come to deny our dependency on others. Rather than embracing dependence and vulnerability, we scorn them as though they are incompatible with autonomy. Kindness, like empathy, inevitably exposes our vulnerability and acknowledges our dependence on others. Darwin argued that we are a profoundly social and caring species, concluding that evolution was not simply a matter of survival of the strongest but the survival of the best adapted, a cohesive group being better adapted for survival (Darwin 2013). Nowadays, in our enterprise culture, practising medicine is often a life of overwork, anxiety and isolation, a culture of competition fostering unkindness. Philips suggests that the joy of kindness is that it opens us to the world of others, the terror

of kindness is that it makes us aware of our own and others vulnera-
bilities (Philips and Taylor 2009). Since vulnerability is an integral part
of kindness and empathy, doctors need to learn to embrace vulnerability rather than pretending that they are omnipotent. In clinical care,
bearing another person's vulnerability means connecting with them and
sharing their suffering without necessarily relieving it. This requires being
able to acknowledge one's own vulnerability. Reflecting on the death
of her father, Palmer wrote "wise decision-making and kindness are not
mentioned in postgraduate medical curriculums yet are at the very root
of clinical practice" (Palmer 2008).

The challenge we face in the West is how do we institutionalise kindness, extend our kindness to family and friends and spread it to meet the
needs of strangers? Philips quotes Winicott, "A sign of health in the mind
is the ability of one individual to enter imaginatively and accurately into
the thoughts and feelings and hopes and fears of another person and also
to allow the other person to do the same to us" (Philips and Taylor 2009).

GENEROSITY

Generosity is the virtue of giving good things to others freely and abun-
dantly (Smith and Davidson 2014). Generosity, a willingness to give of
oneself, is also related to empathy and may be manifest in several ways
in clinical practice: openness to others, providing comfort and a commitment to not abandoning the patient (Frank 2004). Generosity can help
to create social solidarity a sense of 'we're in this together' (Herzog
2020). Individual generosity may rest on a sense of self-transcendence,
a value that can lead people to focus beyond themselves in promoting the
well-being of others (Herzog 2020).

Frank sees generosity beginning in a welcome, as an initial promise
of consolation (Frank 2004). He conceptualises generosity as a capacity
for dialogue, our feeling of being chosen to respond to the suffering of
another person and a sense of gratitude for this privilege (Frank 2004).
Frank identifies a tension between medicine's historic commitment to
hospitality and its current organisation as a business. If instead of thinking
of our duties to others, we think of ourselves, we risk losing a moral vision
of our obligations. In the process of care lies an opportunity for people
to connect and establish a relationship with each other. Patients and their
doctors can feel lonely in the absence of generosity. Verghese expresses a
doctor's perspective:

Despite all our grand societies, memberships, fellowships, speciality colleges, each with its annual dues and certificates and ceremonies, we are horribly alone. The doctor's world is one where our own feelings-particularly those of pain and hurt-are not easily expressed, even though patients are encouraged to express them. We trust our colleagues, we show propriety and reciprocity, we have scientific knowledge, we learn empathy, but we rarely expose our own emotions. (Verghese 1998)

Generosity involves reflecting on patient's stories and in a dialogue finding how to live with disability, illness and suffering (Frank 2004). In a dialogue the doctor talks *with* the patient rather than at them, it involves a sharing of perspective: empathy.

Generosity is the virtue of giving, of going the extra mile, the opposite of selfishness (Comte-Sponville 1996). It has a moral value in avoiding the pettiness of egoism. Generosity can be motivated by solidarity, our relations with others and reflects our interdependence. Descartes proposed generosity as the supreme virtue since to be generous is to be free of self (Descartes 1985).

Generosity aims to enhance the well-being of those to whom something is being given. Generous people can give many things: money, possessions, time, attention, aid, encouragement and emotional availability (Smith and Davidson 2014). In medical practice, giving time is a valuable commodity with which to measure generosity (Huecker 2015).

The paradox of generosity, and in a sense of empathy, is that in giving we receive. In letting go of some of what we own, we better secure our own lives and by giving of ourselves we flourish. The converse is that in being selfish and by failing to care for others, we do not properly take care of ourselves (Smith and Davidson 2014). Smith suggests that people can *learn* generosity and practice it, by first adopting new behaviours that are generous and then reflecting upon their meaning and consequences (Smith and Davidson 2014). Generosity like empathy and other virtues must be practised.

HUMILITY

Humility is another elusive construct; it is not a virtue that doctors claim, to do so would suggest arrogance, the opposite of humility (Murdoch 2013). Western culture celebrates individuality, celebrity, success and competition, where humility may appear unfashionable (Inge 2014).

Humility is derived from the Latin *humus* = ground, to be humble is to be grounded. Humility may be defined as 'a lowly self-opinion; modesty or meekness' ("Chambers 21st Century Dictionary," 1996). However, this narrow definition does not capture the complexity and value of this virtue. Humility requires us to value our own worth appropriately while accepting our helplessness, fallibility and moral frailty and acknowledging our relative insignificance in the universe (Wright 2019).

We perceive the world from our own point of view, often prioritising our own needs and desires. In ethical clinical practice, we need to override this egoism and remove bias. Humility provides a means of achieving this difficult goal (Wright 2019). It allows a doctor to engage with a patient, acknowledging that their needs are as worthy of consideration as her own. Humility, like empathy, is a relational construct which varies in differing contexts and times (Jeffrey 2017; Mosher et al. 2019). In adopting an other-orientated focus, humility moderates the power differences between a doctor and her patient. A humble approach protects us from a narcissistic sense of entitlement which can lead to the disrespectful treatment of a patient or colleague (Wright 2019).

Commonly cited features of humility include self-awareness, openness to possibility and acknowledgement of one's limitations (Tangney 2000). Humility protects us from feelings of entitlement and arrogance. Humility is of particular value when a doctor's beliefs or values are challenged by cultural differences. Humility promotes solidarity and teamworking by reminding us that we all share the same flawed human nature (Wielenberg 2019).

Humility, like empathy and kindness, is a construct which connects doctors and patients (Jeffrey 2016b). In situations of stress, the humble doctor maintains her other-orientated perspective and so promotes positive emotions in the patient (Mosher et al. 2019). Wright suggests that a person with humility is able to escape their own self-centredness and bias to experience the pull of the other's needs as strongly as their own (Wright 2019). Humility leads to a deep connection and a sense of responsibility for others.

Conclusion

This chapter has explored the close relationship between empathy, compassion, sympathy, kindness, generosity and humility. Reflecting on meaningful health outcomes, Palmer suggests two questions which every doctor should ask themselves: "Did I hear what really matters most for this patient right now?" and "Was I kind" (Palmer 2008). A relational conceptualisation of empathy embraces these outcomes and is best suited for medical practice, education and research. Relational empathy forms the core of empathy-based ethics, an approach for ethical practice. The next chapter investigates the process of empathising in the context of the patient-doctor relationship.

REFERENCES

(1996). *Chambers 21st century dictionary.* M. Robinson. Edinburgh: Chambers Harrap.

Ballatt, J., & Campling, P. (2011). *Intelligent kindness.* London: RCPsych Publications.

Batson, C. D. (2011). These things called empathy: Eight related but distinct phenomena. In J. Decety & W. Ickes (Eds.), *The social neuroscience of empathy* (pp. 6–15). Cambridge: MIT Press.

Batson, C. D., et al. (1995). Information function of empathic emotion: Learning that we value the other's welfare. *Journal of Personality and Social Psychology, 68*(2), 300.

Charlton, R. (2016). *Compassion continuity and caring in the NHS.* London: RCGP.

Comte-Sponville, A. (1996). *A short treatise on the great virtues.* London: William Heinemann.

Darwin, C. (2013). *The descent of man.* London: Wordsworth Editions.

Decety, J., et al. (2010). Physicians down-regulate their pain empathy response: An event-related brain potential study. *Neuroimage, 50*(4), 1676–1682.

Descartes, R. (1985). *The philosophical writings of Descartes.* Cambridge: Cambridge University Press.

de Zulueta, P. (2013). Compassion in 21st century medicine: Is it sustainable? *Clinical Ethics, 8*(4), 119–128.

de Zulueta, P. C. (2015). Suffering, compassion and 'doing good medical ethics'. *Journal of Medical Ethics, 41*(1), 87–90.

Francis, R. (2013). *Report of the Mid Staffordshire NHS Foundation Trust public inquiry: Executive summary.* London: HMSO.

Frank, A. (2004). *The renewal of generosity.* Chicago: University of Chicago Press.

Gilbert, P. (2009). *The compassionate mind.* London: Robinson.

Gladkova, A. (2010). Sympathy, compassion and empathy in English and Russian: A linguistic and cultural analysis. *Culture & Psychology, 16*(2), 267–285.

Halpern, J. (2001). *From detached concern to empathy: Humanizing medical practice.* Oxford: Oxford University Press.

Haskins, G., & Thomas, M. (2018). Kindness and its many manifestations. In G. Haskins, M. Thomas, & L. Johri (Eds.), *Kindness in leadership.* London: Routledge.

Herzog, P. S. (2020). *The science of generosity: From disparate to integrated.* Cham: Palgrave Macmillan.

Hojat, M., et al. (2009). The devil is in the third year: A longitudinal study of erosion of empathy in medical school. *Academic Medicine, 84*(9), 1182–1191.

Hojat, M., et al. (2001). The Jefferson scale of physician empathy: Development and preliminary psychometric data. *Educational and Psychological Measurement, 61*(2), 349–365.

Huecker, M. R. (2015). Generosity. *Annals of Emergency Medicine, 65,* 600–601.

Inge, D. (2014). *A tour of bones.* London: Bloomsbury.

Jeffrey, D. (2016a). Clarifying empathy: The first step to more humane clinical care. *British Journal of General Practice, 66,* 101–102.

Jeffrey, D. (2016b). A duty of kindness. *Journal of the Royal Society of Medicine, 109*(7), 261–263.

Jeffrey, D. (2017). Communicating with a human voice: Developing a relational model of empathy. *Journal of the Royal College of Physicians of Edinburgh, 47*(3), 267.

Kohut, H. (1984). *How does analysis cure?* Chicago: University of Chicago Press.

Maxwell, B. (2008). *Professional ethics education: Studies in compassionate empathy.* New York: Springer.

Mercer, S. W., & Reynolds, W. J. (2002). Empathy and quality of care. *British Journal of General Practice, 52,* S9–S12.

Mosher, D. K., et al. (2019). A relational humility framework. In J. C. Wright (Ed.), *Humility.* Oxford: Oxford University Press.

Murdoch, I. (2013). *The sovereignty of good.* London: Routledge.

Palmer, E. (2008). The kindness of strangers. *BMJ, 337,* a1993.

Philips, A., & Taylor, B. (2009). *On kindness.* London: Hamish Hamilton.

Smajdor, A., et al. (2011). The limits of empathy: Problems in medical education and practice. *Journal of Medical Ethics, 37*(6), 380–383.

Smith, C., & Davidson, H. (2014). *The paradox of generosity: Giving we receive, grasping we lose.* Oxford: Oxford University Press.

Stepien, K. A., & Baernstein, A. (2006). Educating for empathy—A review. *Journal of General Internal Medicine, 21*(5), 524–530.

Tangney, J. P. (2000). Humbling: Theoretical perspectives, empirical facts and directions for future research. *Journal of Social and Clinical Psychology, 19,* 70–82.

Verghese, A. (1998). *The tennis partner: A doctor's story of friendship and loss.* New York: Harper Collins.

Warmington, S. (2012). Practising engagement: Infusing communication with empathy and compassion in medical students' clinical encounters. *Health, 16*(3), 327–342.

Wielenberg, E. J. (2019). Secular humility. In J. C. Wright (Ed.), *Humility*. Oxford: Oxford University Press.

Wispé, L. (1986). The distinction between sympathy and empathy: To call forth a concept, a word is needed. *Journal of Personality and Social Psychology, 50*(2), 314.

Wright, J. C. (2019). *Humility*. Oxford: Oxford University Press.

CHAPTER 5

Experiencing Empathy in the Patient-Doctor Relationship

Abstract A partnership model of the patient-doctor relationship involves sharing of information, emotions and decision-making but also sharing of responsibilities. Empathy involves establishing a relationship between the patient and doctor that addresses the patient's psychological and social needs and engages with their suffering. Relational empathy in the patient-doctor relationship is interpreted as an experience between two people and varies according to the context of their meeting. Empathising comprises a series of steps which interact in a subtle psychological dance: concern, attentiveness, sharing emotions, vulnerability, imagination, understanding, dialogue, reflection, authenticity and continuity. Empathy is both a motivating force and a commitment to practical action, responding to suffering. Doctors need support in enhancing their empathic skills. As empathy develops, practice becomes more patient-centred. In conceptualising empathy in a dynamic relational way, doctors are adopting a phenomenological approach to practice by engaging with the experience of the patient.

Keywords Patient-doctor relationship · Empathising · Phenomenology · Emotions · Suffering

43

INTRODUCTION

The central relationship in medical practice is the one between patient and doctor. The quality of this relationship may affect the content of the communication between them and so affect the outcome of medical practice. It is beyond the scope of this book to review the many differing models of the patient-doctor relationship, ranging from physician-centred paternalistic models to patient-centred consumerist ones. The type of model most applicable to an empathic relationship is a mutual partnership model, in which power is equally distributed between patient and doctor, and goals are negotiated in a dialogue in which the patient's values and feelings are explored. The ethical process of informed consent is central to this relationship (Marcum 2008). A partnership model stresses sharing of information, emotions and decision-making but also a sharing of responsibilities by both the doctor and the patient. The patient-doctor relationship involves two individuals with differing concerns but sharing the same aim, the well-being of the patient (Mallia 2013). Empathy involves the establishment of a relationship between the patient and doctor that addresses the patient's psychological and social needs and engages with suffering (Marcum 2008).

Quantitative research describes empathy as a static attribute, a possession, which the doctor either has or does not have (Hojat et al. 2009). This intrapersonal view of empathy underpins the theory behind most of the research directed at measuring empathy (Hojat et al. 2009). However, this static view of empathy fails to clarify how it is experienced and disregards the impact of context (Campos et al. 2011; Marshall and Hooker 2016).

In contrast, this chapter examines relational empathy in the context of the patient-doctor relationship. Empathy is interpreted as an experience between two people and varies according to the context of their meeting (Jeffrey 2017). C. Batson (2011) captured the complexity of empathy by identifying eight related but distinct phenomena which are described as 'empathies' in the literature. His description of eight 'empathies' conveniently summarises the complexity of empathy before the process of empathising with another person is explored:

1. Knowing another person's internal state, including thoughts and feelings: sometimes described as cognitive empathy (Wispé 1986).

2. Adopting the posture of an observed other: motor mimicry (Lipps 1903).
3. Coming to feel as another person feels: affective empathy, emotional contagion or sympathy (Hoffman 2000).
4. Projecting oneself into another's situation: an aesthetic projection described as *Einfühlung* (Lipps 1903).
5. Imaging how another is thinking or feeling: other-orientated perspective taking (Batson et al. 1991).
6. Imagining how one would think and feel in the other's place: self-orientated perspective taking (Batson et al. 1997).
7. Feeling distress at witnessing another's suffering, personal distress (Batson and Shaw 1991).
8. Feeling for another person who is suffering, empathic concern (Batson 2011).

Batson's eight phenomena, each a form of empathy, provide a helpful basis for investigating the process of empathising (Batson 2011). The first six concepts are related to the question of how we know another person's thoughts. The last two concepts (concepts 7 and 8) are reactions to this knowledge, reflecting a caring response to suffering. It is not only other-orientated feelings (concept 8) which are a source of a caring response. A sensitive response may result from feeling as the other (concept 3), combined with an other-orientated perspective (concept 5) (Batson 2011).

In discussing the process of empathy in the context of clinical practice, the debate moves beyond arguments over how this complex concept should be defined into deeper thinking about the nature of the patient-doctor relationship (Coplan and Goldie 2011; Irving and Dickson 2004; Marshall and Hooker 2016). Empathy is often described in the literature as something which occurs between a doctor and a patient but not as something which is influenced by time, stress or the culture of the organisation (Marshall and Hooker 2016). A relational view of empathy is less concerned with what characteristics the doctor 'has', but rather focuses on what happens in the patient-doctor relationship: the process of empathising (Marshall and Hooker 2016).

EMPATHISING: A DYNAMIC RELATIONAL PROCESS

Empathy is a dynamic process where both patient and doctor learn more about each other over time in an iterative deepening of their relationship(Barrett-Lennard 1981). Empathising comprises a series of steps which interact, according to the context of the relationship, in a subtle psychological dance. Interrogating the process may help to address the empathy gap which exists in practice and so to develop more humane care.

EMPATHIC CONCERN

Empathy begins with an individual's willingness and capacity to empathise (Uygur et al. 2019). This initial concern or 'empathic resonation' between a doctor and patient ensures that empathy is an interpersonal phenomenon from the outset (Barrett-Lennard 1981; Håkansson and Montgomery 2003). Suchman describes this moment as 'empathic opportunity' (Suchman et al. 1997). Doctors want to empathise with patients and feel frustrated when prevented from doing so (Howick et al. 2018; Tavakol et al. 2012). The empathic doctor tries to see the world through the patient's eyes using imagination and curiosity. Letting go of assumptions forms part of our willingness to empathise. The doctor may adopt Carl Roger's therapeutic stance of 'unconditional positive regard' for the patient (Rogers 1995).

Appropriate empathic concern should be distinguished from personal distress which may result from over-identifying with the patient (Decety and Lamm 2011). Stress may result from taking a self-orientated perspective (how would I feel in this situation?) which can lead to identification and becoming overwhelmed.

ATTENTIVENESS

Attentiveness involves a doctor's openness both to the patient's feelings and to their own emotions (Warmington 2012). Empathy can be enhanced by simply being present, by giving the other person the focus of one's full attention. A deep level of empathy requires face-to-face contact with the other person and cannot occur while the doctor is gazing at a computer screen. Attention involves active listening as a doctor seeks the underlying hidden agenda each patient brings, listening to their story and giving them time.

SHARING EMOTIONS

Doctors struggle in their relationships with patients to balance emotional connection and detached professional concern (Hojat et al. 2009; Halpern 2001; Weatherall 1994). The GMC publishes ethical advice on maintaining a professional boundary between a doctor and patient: "You must not use your professional position to pursue a sexual or improper emotional relationship with a patient or someone close to them" (General Medical Council 2013). While improper emotional relationships are prohibited, a proper close empathic relationship with a patient encourages trust, allowing patients to confide their deepest fears. Empathy involves feeling with the patient to gain an understanding of their suffering (Svenaeus 2015).

McNaughton asks, 'Where has the idea originated that to be a good doctor one must remove emotion from reason, or so dilute it for the patient's benefit, to result in detached concern?' (McNaughton 2013). Patients want their doctors to demonstrate empathic concern (Mercer and Reynolds 2002). Empathic concern results in a sharing of emotion; the doctor feels the pain of a patient while, at the same time, remaining aware of the self-other boundary (Decety and Ickes 2011). In this way, doctors can become aware of the quality of the patient's emotion without its potentially overwhelming intensity. Agosta (2014) supported this view by claiming that in empathy, the doctor takes a sample of the suffering of the patient without over-identifying with the other person. Emotionally engaged doctors communicate more effectively with patients (Girgis and Sanson-Fisher 1995; Halpern 2014; Kim et al. 2004; Kozlowski et al. 2017). Emotions enable a doctor to focus on their work and should be used by the doctor to guide their responses in a particular context (Gillies and Sheehan 2005).

Doctors may fear emotional connection because they are concerned that their clinical judgement may be less 'objective', or that they will become overwhelmed and suffer burnout. Burnout, a stress-related syndrome, is characterised by exhaustion, depersonalisation and a diminished sense of accomplishment, and is related to lower empathy (Brazeau et al. 2010; Thomas et al. 2007). These concerns may lead them to distance themselves from patients, mistakenly feeling that detachment is part of being professional. However, empathic doctors have more job satisfaction and less burnout than detached colleagues (Kearney et al. 2009; Sturzu et al. 2019; Zenasni et al. 2012). Even if doctors try to suppress their feelings by distancing themselves, they cannot avoid having emotional attitudes towards patients (Larson and Yao 2005).

The idea that emotions are disruptive, and need to be controlled, is deeply ingrained in medical education and practice (Montgomery 2006). A recent review demonstrated that emotions contributed to clinical decisions, concluding that they played an integral part in patient safety (Heyhoe et al. 2016).

VULNERABILITY

Doctors face the challenge of being open with patients while accepting their own vulnerability, without distancing or necessarily trying to 'fix things'. Empathy inevitably exposes our vulnerability and involves sharing part of oneself with the other person (Krznaric 2014). If we are to bridge the empathy gap, we need to develop a medical culture which acknowledges the doctor's vulnerability. It is easy to forget how effective it is simply allowing a patient to talk, express emotions or cry (Connelly 2009).

Ricoeur explored the connection between vulnerability and empathy. He argued that although there are differences between people we are bound together in a search for mutual recognition and understanding (Ricoeur 1992). He claimed that we are simultaneously capable and vulnerable, blurring role boundaries that assigned competence to doctors and vulnerability to patients. Selfhood and otherness cannot be separated, to be able to see oneself as another implies being able to see another as oneself, so the suffering of others becomes our suffering (Ricoeur 1992).

The power differences between doctor and patient are reminiscent of Foucault's concept of 'the gaze' which described medical ways of knowing that put the doctor in the position of an observer of the patient and their disease (Bleakley and Bligh 2009). This positioning objectifies the patient, making them a passive source of scientific interest and is dehumanising (Marshall and Hooker 2016). Shapiro argues that if working out how to bridge the inevitable distance between a doctor and a patient is at the heart of good medical practice, then empathy is the most important of the professional virtues (Shapiro 2008).

EMOTIONAL REGULATION: BALANCING CONNECTION AND DETACHMENT

Doctors often struggle to achieve an appropriate balance between detachment from and connection with a patient. A self-other boundary is needed which permits emotional engagement yet prevents the doctor becoming overwhelmed by distress. Frank described the idea of alterity, involving a recognition of the other person as being separate from oneself, allowing the possibility of genuine dialogue and true empathy (Frank 2004). In an empathic relationship, both the doctor and the patient are enabled to have a voice, and in so doing, their alterity is respected (Frank 2004). Bondi developed these ideas by suggesting alterity was an unconscious process in which the doctor was both a subjectively engaged participant in a two-person relationship and at the same time an observer of that relationship. This 'third position' allowed the doctor to be subjectively absorbed in the patient's narrative as well as maintaining a capacity to step back and reflect on that absorption (Bondi 2014).

Taking an other-orientated perspective is part of forming a psychological boundary with the other person, resonating with Rogers' work. He claimed that although empathy should involve a deep engagement with the patient, it did not mean that the doctor loses sight of where the self ends and the other begins. He stressed that empathy involves entering the perceived world of the other person 'as if' one were the other person, but without ever losing the 'as if' condition (Rogers 1959). Rogers' account conceptualises empathy as an experience which paradoxically combines closeness and distance, similarity and difference (Bondi 2008). Empathy creates a space which enables the doctor and patient to convey respect and recognition (Bondi 2003). In empathy, the doctor is emotionally engaged with the patient and at same time she is reflecting on these emotions, knowing that they originate in the other person (Halpern 2001).

To maintain this delicate psychological balance between detachment and connection, the doctor needs to be self-aware, to reflect on their work and to have access to support. A self-aware doctor understands that her own feelings and the part they play in the consultation are an integral part of her empathy (Balint 1957; Bondi 2014).

IMAGINATION

Empathy involves using one's imagination, which can be self or other orientated. In taking a self-orientated perspective, I imagine what it is like for me to be in your situation, a form of identification (Bondi 2014). Doctors who take a self-orientated perspective are at risk not only of personal distress, but compassion fatigue and eventually burnout (Kearney et al. 2009). In contrast, taking an other-orientated perspective, as in relational empathy, involves imagining undergoing the patient's experience and is essential for appropriate empathetic concern. This more sophisticated approach requires mental flexibility and an ability to regulate one's emotions. Taking an other-orientated perspective prevents the doctor from losing sight of the patient as another person, despite having a deep engagement with them (Coplan and Goldie 2011; Rogers 1961).

UNDERSTANDING

The patient and doctor engage in a construction of meaning through interpretation, an iterative process, to gain understanding (Hooker 2015). While I argue for adopting emotional-based reasoning instead of detached concern, the cognitive dimension of empathy is a core element of empathy. In the 'detached concern' form of empathising, understanding occurs within the doctor. In contrast, in a relational model, understanding is an interpersonal activity depending on the doctor and the patient who also gains an understanding of the doctor's world. Doctors need 'narrative competency' to allow them to interact with the patient in a joint process of making sense of their stories of suffering (Charon 2001). Empathy cannot achieve an identical or complete understanding of the other person but in reaching out and connecting with the other and accounting for differences in perspectives empathy can be of great value.

RESPECTFUL DIALOGUE

Empathy has a moral dimension, since appropriate understanding of the patient is necessary before being in a position to respond in an ethical way (Pedersen 2008). The doctor and patient participate in a dialogue and reflect on their understanding. Frank suggests that it is at precisely the moment when two people share feelings of uncertainty, vulnerability and loneliness that dialogue is most possible between them (Frank 2004). A respectful dialogue is one in which each of the participants is able to voice their separate viewpoints (Warmington 2012). Respectful dialogue entails reciprocal and iterative acts of attention, representation and interpretation (Charon 2006).

Dostoevsky describes such a moment in *The Possessed:*

> We are two human beings, and have come together in infinity for the last time in the world. Drop your tone, and speak like a human being! Speak, if only for once in your life, with the voice of a man. (Dostovesky 1952)

Dialogue is a powerful way of connecting with patients and overcomes the distancing that demoralises both the doctor and the patient. Empathy can be seen as a dynamic emotional resonance: a dialogue between a patient and a doctor (Warmington 2012). The moral demand of a dialogue is that each participant grants equal authority to the other's voice, speaking *with* the other rather that speaking *about* them (Frank 2004).

Empathy is a source of moral knowledge and an essential component of practical wisdom (*phronesis*) and of empathy-based ethics (Chochinov 2007; Noddings 1984). Medical practice involves a flow of ethical decisions between doctor and patient; at its heart, medicine is a moral endeavour (Frank 2004).

COMMUNICATION

Non-verbal communication skills include eye contact, touch, facial expression and other body language communicating concern. Reflecting the patient's feeling is an important verbal tool in conveying empathy along with the sensitive use of language and self-disclosure (Irving and Dickson 2004). Empathy provides a space for engaging with the patient and resolving problems in an ongoing interactive process, what was previously unknown is revealed by combining understanding, interpretation and listening (Agosta 2014). To fully understand another person's experience does sometimes require direct enquiry, at other times silence, while maintaining a presence, may be a more appropriate response.

AUTHENTICITY

Authentic empathic engagement affirms the patient's strengths, accepts weaknesses and is non-judgemental (Charon 2001). At one end of a spectrum of empathy, medical students describe 'fake' empathy in OSCE exams where they show empathic behaviours without trying to understand the patient's view (Jeffrey 2018). Jamison highlighted the difference between a student being assessed for empathy and the nuanced nature of true empathy in practice (Jamison 2014). Fake empathy has been compared to surface acting in which empathic expressions are adopted without any change in the student's emotions or understanding of the patient (Larson and Yao 2005). The next level of empathy is 'detached concern' which does not attempt to make an emotional connection with the patient (Halpern 2001). Agosta takes a stronger position by dismissing detached concern as being a professionally motivated lack of empathy (Agosta 2014).

In contrast, authentic relational empathy seems similar to deep acting where the actor feels the emotions rather than merely altering their emotional expressions (Larson and Yao 2005). Larson claimed that the scope of empathy goes far beyond the communication skills of surface acting (Larson and Yao 2005). True relational empathy involves connecting with the patient both cognitively and emotionally, acting to help the patient with a feeling of responsibility for their care (Macintyre 1985). True empathy is not only a sharing of feelings and understanding, but it is also a way of responding to the patient (Svenaeus 2015). Empathy conceptualised at this level involves recognition of the patient as a fellow human being and developing a sense of fraternity. This feeling of a shared humanity can create a sense of security in situations of great uncertainty, for instance, in end-of-life care (Svenaeus 2014).

REFLECTION

Reflection is central to empathising, developing with experience from a conscious reflection on experience, through reflection in action, to a way of being, of a mindful practice (Johns 2017). An ethical pause to reflect on a wider picture, accounting for the context and for psychosocial aspects of the patient's world, integrating the objective and subjective, is necessary before reaching decisions. Reflecting on one's experience and feelings provides a doctor with fresh insights and enables them to be open to new possibilities. Reflection in the context of an empathic relationship facilitates connection and so eases suffering (Johns 2017).

In reflecting on experience, a doctor can acknowledge their emotions and so improve their clinical effectiveness as well as their well-being (Connelly 2009). It is through reflection that a doctor achieves sound judgement or *phronesis* (practical wisdom). In reflecting on their experiences, a doctor recognises their own limitations and learns to tolerate uncertainty. Providing doctors with time and space for reflection, mentoring and support may foster empathy (Lutz et al. 2013).

CONTINUITY

A relational view of empathy implies that the doctor's success in empathising with a patient partially depended on the openness of patient and on the context of their meeting (Halpern 2001; Main et al. 2017). Feedback from the patient can help a doctor to develop a greater understanding of the patient's lifeworld (Main et al. 2017). Empathy as a relational concept deepens with continuity of care (Sulzer et al. 2016). Continuity of care is difficult to achieve in the UK nowadays as many patients feel that they cannot relate to 'their' general practitioner as they see different doctors each time they visit the surgery (Charlton 2016).

COMMITMENT TO ACTION

Motivation to act is thought by some authors to be a feature of compassion which differentiates it from empathy (Chochinov 2007). However, empathy is both a motivating force and a commitment to practical action, thus moving beyond Batson's empathy-altruism hypothesis towards a view of empathy as a response to suffering (Batson 2011; Warmington 2012). Expanding the concept of empathy to include action to relieve suffering maintains the focus on the patient rather than the doctor and takes account of the social context of the patient's illness (Garden 2009). Recognising a patient's suffering was a starting point for empathy with action, in which a doctor explores the patient's experience of illness and their social situation, before acting with them to alleviate suffering (Garden 2009). The nature of the commitment between doctor and patient will depend on context; in many cases, it will be to ease suffering; in other situations, it may be to make a diagnosis, or not to abandon the patient (Warmington 2012).

SUPPORT

Doctors need support in enhancing their empathic skills. Stress may inhibit emotional engagement and that conversely support, which reduces stress, allowed doctors to be more open to emotions (Marshall and Hooker 2016). Doctors need to develop the self-awareness to recognise the difference between empathic concern which is an essential part of professionalism, and personal distress, which can be self-destructive. However, it is not good enough to provide doctors with training or exhortations to be more empathic and then expect them to work in an environment which does not support empathy. Support needs to be available for all doctors and medical students not just reserved for those perceived to be struggling (Jeffrey 2014).

CONTEXT

Relational empathy is affected by the physical context of the meeting between patient and doctor. Interruptions, lack of privacy and consultations at the bedside in a group setting are common constraints in a hospital setting (Warmington 2012). Patients express a preference for personalised care from a doctor whom they know and trust (Bensing et al. 2013). Collaborative multidisciplinary teamwork is an integral part of the context of modern clinical practice but may lead to a dilution of responsibility which leaves the patient feeling abandoned by the doctor (Bleakley and Bligh 2009). Relational empathy depends upon both the patient and the doctor in a relationship which may be challenged by a variety of factors including: lack of time, continuity, stress and a culture focused on technical efficiency. Attributes of the patient and the doctor may affect the consultation: gender, educational level and ethnicity (Warmington 2012).

It could be questioned whether it is reasonable to expect doctors to have empathetic relationships with patients given the demands of medical practice in the NHS today. Shortage of time may lead to a neglect of psychosocial issues and to medical errors. Considerations of efficiency have largely superseded personalised patient care (Derksen et al. 2020).

It is possible that spending time with patients, listening and carefully examining them might avoid unnecessary tests and procedures (Howick et al. 2020). While fast medicine is appropriate in emergency situations, there may be a place for slow medicine in many of the illnesses which evolve chronically (Bauer 2008). Authors have also described a 'slow medical education' where instead of a rush to efficiency, there was a commitment by the faculty to provide time for students to reflect about their experiences (Wear et al. 2014).

Another possible factor in the dehumanising of doctors and students is the transient nature of relationships during training where temporary relationships lacking in human connection both with patients and with colleagues result in a pressure to do something. In this way, 'efficient' doctors may become alienated from patients and doctors who do spend time with patients risk being regarded as inefficient (Christakis and Feudtner 1997).

Finally, it can be argued that allowing the patient to create a narrative is not as time-consuming as may be assumed (Hardy 2017). It has been shown that allowing a patient to establish their story takes approximately two minutes, for 78% of those patients (Langewitz et al. 2002). However, on average, doctors interrupt the patient's story after a mean of 23 seconds (Marvel et al. 1999). There is therefore scope for doctors who possess 'narrative competence' to allow patients to complete their story in a short time within an empathic relationship.

Doctors tend to distance themselves from patients when they felt stressed, reducing empathy and increasing the risk of clinical errors and further stress (Ahrweiler et al. 2014). Strategies for coping with stress that involved detachment from the patients correlate with depression, anxiety and poor mental health. In contrast, strategies that involved engagement, support and expression of emotion enabled doctors to respond in a healthy way (Dyrbye et al. 2005).

Conclusions

Twenty years ago, Jodi Halpern, in her seminal work, *From Detached Concern to Empathy; Humanizing Medical Practice*, suggested that doctors should adopt a model of empathy which included affective dimensions instead of detached concern (Halpern 2001). I echo her plea and argue that by analysing the process of empathising a broad model of empathy emerges, moving beyond detached concern to a dynamic relational approach. In this approach, empathising becomes a creative process which changes and develops with experience. As empathy develops, practice becomes more patient-centred. If doctors are to establish close therapeutic relationships with patients, they need to be given time to establish empathy, to acknowledge the individuality of the patient and to properly address their concerns (Howie et al. 1999). Time, presence, feelings, curiosity and imagination combine in empathy to recognise the person not simply their illness.

In conceptualising empathy in a dynamic relational way, doctors are adopting a phenomenological approach to practice by engaging with the experience of the patient (Hooker 2015). Phenomenology aims at gaining a deeper understanding of the meaning of our everyday, taken-for-granted, experiences as they are lived (Van Manen 2016). It can also be described as a way of seeing how things appear to us through experience, from an individual's perspective (Carel 2016; Finlay 2013; Smith et al. 2009). Such a process of active connection with the experiences of another person is central to empathy and to phenomenology (Main et al. 2017). Empathy becomes a special form of understanding and extends to become a way of being. Hooker proposes that "empathy is one of the key hallmarks of good doctoring" (Hooker 2015). A willingness to feel and convey empathy may result in a culture shift in medicine from detached concern to a broader relational view of empathy as the appropriate way of seeing the world from the patient's point of view.

Halpern maintains that empathy elevates a doctor's work from just a job to a profession in which she contributes to the meaningfulness of people's lives (Halpern 2001). Perhaps every doctor, clinical teacher and medical student needs to ask themselves "Do I speak with a human voice ?".

REFERENCES

Agosta, L. (2014). A rumor of empathy: Reconstructing Heidegger's contribution to empathy and empathic clinical practice. *Medicine, Health Care and Philosophy, 17*(2), 281–292.

Ahrweiler, F., et al. (2014). Determinants of physician empathy during medical education: Hypothetical conclusions from an exploratory qualitative survey of practicing physicians. *BMC Medical Education, 14,* 122–134.

Balint, M. (1957). *The doctor his patient and the illness*. London: Tavistock Publications.

Barrett-Lennard, G. T. (1981). The empathy cycle: Refinement of a nuclear concept. *Journal of Counseling Psychology, 28*(2), 91–100.

Batson, C. D. (2011). These things called empathy: Eight related but distinct phenomena. In J. Decety & W. Ickes (Eds.), *The social neuroscience of empathy* (pp. 6–15). Cambridge: MIT Press.

Batson, C. D., et al. (1991). Empathic joy and the empathy-altruism hypothesis. *Journal of Personality and Social Psychology, 61*(3), 413–426.

Batson, C. D., et al. (1997). Perspective taking: Imagining how another feels versus imaging how you would feel. *Personality and Social Psychology Bulletin, 23*(7), 751–758.

Batson, C. D., & Shaw, L. L. (1991). Evidence for altruism: Toward a pluralism of prosocial motives. *Psychological Inquiry, 2*(2), 107–122.

Bauer, J. L. (2008). Slow medicine. *The Journal of Alternative and Complementary Medicine, 14*, 891–892.

Bensing, J., et al. (2013). What patients want. *Patient Education and Counseling, 90*, 287–290.

Bleakley, A., & Bligh, J. (2009). Who can resist Foucault? *Journal of Medicine and Philosophy, 34*(4), 368–383.

Bondi, L. (2003). Empathy and identification: Conceptual resources for feminist fieldwork. *ACME: An International E-Journal for Critical Geographies, 2*(1), 64–76.

Bondi, L. (2008). On the relational dynamics of caring: A psychotherapeutic approach to emotional and power dimensions of women's care work. *Gender, Place and Culture, 15*(3), 249–265.

Bondi, L. (2014). Understanding feelings: Engaging with unconscious communication and embodied knowledge. *Emotion, Space and Society, 10*, 44–54.

Brazeau, C., et al. (2010). Relationships between medical student burnout, empathy, and professionalism climate. *Academic Medicine, 85*(10), 33–36.

Campos, J. J., et al. (2011). Reconceptualizing emotion regulation. *Emotion Review, 3*(1), 26–35.

Carel, H. (2016). *The phenomenology of illness*. Oxford: Oxford University Press.

Charlton, R. (2016). *Compassion, continuity and caring in the NHS*. London: RCGP.

Charon, R. (2001). Narrative medicine—A model for empathy, reflection, profession, and trust. *Journal of the American Medical Association, 286*(15), 1897–1902.

Charon, R. (2006). *Narrative medicine: Honoring the stories of illness*. New York: Oxford University Press.

Chochinov, H. (2007). Dignity and the essence of medicine: The A, B, C, and D of dignity conserving care. *BMJ, 335*, 184–187.

Christakis, D., & Feudtner, C. (1997). Temporary matters: The ethical consequences of transient social relationships in medical training. *Journal of the American Medical Association, 278*(9), 739–743.

Connelly, J. E. (2009). The avoidance of human suffering. *Perspectives in Biology and Medicine, 52*, 381–391.

Coplan, A., & Goldie, P. (Eds.). (2011). *Empathy: Philosophical and psychological perspectives*. Oxford: Oxford University Press.

Decety, J., & Ickes, W. (2011). *The social neuroscience of empathy.* Cambridge: MIT Press.

Decety, J., & Lamm, C. (2011). Empathy versus personal distress: Recent evidence from social neuroscience. In J. Decety & W. Ickes (Eds.), *The social neuroscience of empathy* (pp. 199–213). Cambridge: MIT Press.

Derksen, F., et al. (2020). The human encounter, attention, and equality: The value of doctor–patient contact. *British Journal of General Practice, 70,* 254–255.

Dostovesky, F. (1952). *The possessed.* London: J &M Dent.

Dyrbye, L. N., et al. (2005). Medical student distress: Causes, consequences and proposed solutions. *Mayo Clinic Proceedings, 80*(12), 1613–1622.

Finlay, L. (2013). Unfolding the phenomenological research process: Iterative stages of "seeing afresh". *Journal of Humanistic Psychology, 53*(2), 172–201.

Frank, A. (2004). *The renewal of generosity.* Chicago: University of Chicago Press.

Garden, R. (2009). Expanding clinical empathy: An activist perspective. *Journal of General Internal Medicine, 24*(1), 122–125.

General Medical Council. (2013). *Good medical practice.* London: General Medical Council.

Gillies, J., & Sheehan, M. (2005). Perceptual capacity and the good GP: Invisible, yet indispensable for quality of care. *British Journal of General Practice, 55*(521), 974–977.

Girgis, A., & Sanson-Fisher, R. W. (1995). Breaking bad news: Consensus guidelines for medical practitioners. *Journal of Clinical Oncology, 13*(9), 2449–2456.

Håkansson, J., & Montgomery, H. (2003). Empathy as an interpersonal phenomenon. *Journal of Social and Personal Relationships, 20*(3), 267–284.

Halpern, J. (2001). *From detached concern to empathy: Humanizing medical practice.* Oxford: Oxford University Press.

Halpern, J. (2014). From idealized clinical empathy to empathic communication in medical care. *Medicine, Health Care and Philosophy, 17*(2), 301–311.

Hardy, C. (2017). Empathizing with patients: The role of interaction and narratives in providing better patient care. *Medicine, Healthcare and Philosophy, 20,* 237–248.

Heyhoe, J., et al. (2016). The role of emotion in patient safety: Are we brave enough to scratch beneath the surface? *Journal of the Royal Society of Medicine, 109*(2), 52–58.

Hoffman, M. L. (2000). *Empathy and moral development: Implications for caring and justice.* Cambridge: Cambridge University Press.

Hojat, M., et al. (2009). The devil is in the third year: A longitudinal study of erosion of empathy in medical school. *Academic Medicine, 84*(9), 1182–1191.

Hooker, C. (2015). Understanding empathy: Why phenomenology and hermeneutics can help medical education and practice. *Medicine, Health Care and Philosophy, 18*(4), 541–552.

Howick, J., et al. (2018). Effects of empathic and positive communication in healthcare consultations: A systematic review and meta-analysis. *Journal of the Royal Society of Medicine, 111,* 240–252.

Howick, J., et al. (2020). A price tag on clinical empathy? Factors influencing its cost-effectiveness. *Journal Royal Society Medicine, 11,* 389.

Howie, J. G., et al. (1999). Quality at general practice consultations: Cross-sectional survey. *BMJ, 319*(7212), 738–743.

Irving, P., & Dickson, D. (2004). Empathy: Towards a conceptual framework for health professionals. *International Journal of Health Care Quality Assurance, 17*(4), 212–220.

Jamison, L. (2014). *The empathy exams.* London: Granta.

Jeffrey, D. (2014). *Medical mentoring: Supporting students, doctors in training and general practitioners.* London: Royal College of General Practitioners.

Jeffrey, D. (2017). Communicating with a human voice: Developing a relational model of empathy. *Journal of the Royal College of Physicians of Edinburgh, 47*(3), 267.

Jeffrey, D. (2018). *Exploring empathy with medical students: A qualitative longitudinal phenomenological study* (PhD thesis). University of Edinburgh.

Johns, C. (2017). *Becoming a reflective practitioner.* Chichester: Wiley Blackwell.

Kearney, M. K., et al. (2009). Self-care of physicians caring for Patients at the end of Life "Being connected....A key to survival". *Journal of the American Medical Association, 301,* 1155–1164.

Kim, S. S., et al. (2004). The effects of physician empathy on patient satisfaction and compliance. *Evaluation and the Health Professions, 27*(3), 237–251.

Kozlowski, D., et al. (2017). The role of emotion in clinical decision making: An integrative literature review. *BMC Medical Education, 17*(1), 255–268.

Krznaric, R. (2014). *Empathy: A handbook for revolution.* London: Random House.

Langewitz, W., et al. (2002). Spontaneous talking time at start of consultation in outpatient clinic: Cohort study. *BMJ, 325*(7366), 682–683.

Larson, E., & Yao, X. (2005). Clinical empathy as emotional labor in the patient-physician relationship. *Journal of the American Medical Association, 293*(9), 1100–1106.

Lipps, T. (1903). *Asthetik.* Leipzig, Germany: Leopold Voss Verlag.

Lutz, G., et al. (2013). A reflective practice intervention for professional development, reduced stress and improved patient care—A qualitative developmental evaluation. *Patient Education and Counseling, 92*(3), 337–345.

Macintyre, A. (1985). *After virtue.* London: Duckworth.

Main, A., et al. (2017). The interpersonal functions of empathy: A relational perspective. *Emotion Review, 9*, 358–366.

Mallia, P. (2013). *The nature of the doctor-patient relationship: Health care principles through the phenomenology of relationships with patients.* Dordrecht: Springer.

Marcum, J. A. (2008). *An introductory philosophy of medicine: Humanizing modern medicine.* Dortrecht: Springer.

Marshall, G. R. E., & Hooker, C. (2016). Empathy and affect: What can empathied bodies do? *Medical Humanities, 42*, 128–134.

Marvel, M. K., et al. (1999). Soliciting the patient's agenda: Have we improved? *Journal of the American Medical Association, 281*(3), 283–287.

McNaughton, N. (2013). Discourse(s) of emotion within medical education: The ever-present absence. *Medical Education, 47*(1), 71–79.

Mercer, S. W., & Reynolds, W. J. (2002). Empathy and quality of care. *British Journal of General Practice, 52*, S9–S12.

Montgomery, K. (2006). *How doctors think: Clinical judgment and the practice of medicine.* Oxford: Oxford University Press.

Noddings, N. (1984). *Caring: A feminine approach to ethics and moral education.* Berkeley: University of California Press.

Pedersen, R. (2008). Empathy: A wolf in sheep's clothing? *Medicine, Health Care and Philosophy, 11*(3), 325–335.

Ricoeur, P. (1992). *Oneself as another.* Chicago: University of Chicago Press.

Rogers, C. R. (1959). A theory of therapy, personality and interpersonal relationships as developed in the client-centered framework. In S. E. Koch (Ed.), *Psychology: A study of science: Formulations of the person and the social context* (Vol. 3). New York: McGraw-Hill.

Rogers, C. R. (1995). *A way of being.* Boston: Houghton Mifflin Harcourt.

Rogers, C. R. (1961). *On becoming a person.* London: Constable.

Shapiro, J. (2008). Walking a mile in their patients' shoes: Empathy and othering in medical students' education. *Philosophy, Ethics, and Humanities in Medicine, 3*, 10–21.

Smith, J. A., et al. (2009). *Interpretative phenomenological analysis: Theory, method and research.* London: Sage.

Sturzu, L., et al. (2019). Empathy and burnout—A cross-sectional study among mental healthcare providers in France. *Journal of Medicine and Life, 12*, 21–29.

Suchman, A. L., et al. (1997). A model of empathic communication in the medical interview. *Journal of the American Medical Association, 277*(8), 678–682.

Sulzer, S. H., et al. (2016). Assessing empathy development in medical education: A systematic review. *Medical Education, 50*(3), 300–310.

Svenaeus, F. (2014). Empathy as a necessary condition of phronesis: A line of thought for medical ethics. *Medicine, Health Care and Philosophy, 17*(2), 293–299.

Svenaeus, F. (2015). The relationship between empathy and sympathy in good health care. *Medicine, Health Care and Philosophy, 18*(2), 267–277.

Tavakol, S., et al. (2012). Medical students' understanding of empathy: A phenomenological study. *Medical Education, 46*(7), 306–316.

Thomas, M. R., et al. (2007). How do distress and well-being relate to medical student empathy? A multicenter study. *Journal of General Internal Medicine, 22*(2), 177–183.

Uygur, J., et al. (2019). Understanding compassion in family medicine: A qualitative study. *British Journal of General Practice, 69*, 208–216.

Van Manen, M. (2016). *Researching lived experience: Human science for an action sensitive pedagogy.* London: Routledge.

Warmington, S. (2012). Practising engagement: Infusing communication with empathy and compassion in medical students' clinical encounters. *Health, 16*(3), 327–342.

Wear, D., et al. (2014). Slow medical education. *Academic Medicine, 90*, 289–293.

Weatherall, D. (1994). The inhumanity of medicine. *BMJ, 309*, 1671.

Wispé, L. (1986). The distinction between sympathy and empathy: To call forth a concept, a word is needed. *Journal of Personality and Social Psychology, 50*(2), 314.

Zenasni, F., et al. (2012). Burnout and empathy in primary care: Three hypotheses. *British Journal of General Practice, 62*(600), 346–347.

CHAPTER 6

The Role of Empathy in Humane Medicine

Abstract Patients want care that explores their concerns, seeks an understanding of their world and their emotional needs within a continuing relationship with their doctors. Empathy is critical for reaching an accurate diagnosis, for effective ethical care which responds to patients and connects with their suffering. Empathy aims to understand both the emotional and cognitive aspects of the patient's concerns well enough to address their medical problems in an appropriate way, to build a therapeutic partnership. The benefits of empathy include improved health outcomes, trust, altruism, patient satisfaction, patient-centred care and enhanced autonomy. Empathy enriches the patient-doctor relationship and reduces physician burnout. Respecting a patient's dignity involves relational empathy in seeing the world from their point of view and communicating to the patient that they matter.

Keywords Aims of empathy · Benefits of empathy · Patient-doctor relationship · Patient-centred care · Relational empathy

INTRODUCTION

There is a broad consensus that empathy is of fundamental importance in clinical medicine (Derksen et al. 2013; Howick et al. 2018). Patients want care that explores their concerns, seeks an understanding of their world and their emotional needs within a continuing relationship with their doctors (Little et al. 2001; Stewart 2001). Empathy is critical for reaching an accurate diagnosis and for effective ethical care; to learn of the patient's subjective feelings, supplementing objective scientific knowledge. Empathy is a fundamental part of a doctor's capacity to respond to patients ethically, not only to connect with their suffering but to respond to it in an appropriate way (Noddings 2013). This chapter outlines the aims of relational empathy and explores the ways in which it leads to more humane practice.

AIMS OF RELATIONAL EMPATHY

Empathy aims to understand both the emotional and cognitive aspects of the patient's concerns well enough to address their medical problems in an appropriate way, to build a therapeutic partnership (Halpern 2014). It encompasses both understanding, emotional sharing and a caring response to the individual patient's concerns. Listening in an attuned way, a core component of empathy, plays an important part in taking a "good history" from the patient. Empathy is essential for doctors interpreting the patient's story in the medical notes as a clinical "history", as there is a risk that patient's voice is lost in a technical description of symptoms and signs of disease. It is vital therefore that doctors can empathise with patients in order to accurately and honestly portray the patient's subjective views and wider concerns in the medical record (Kim et al. 2004). In addition to the aims of facilitating communication, increasing understanding and improving decision-making, empathy plays a core ethical role in identifying and addressing moral issues in the patient's story (Maxwell 2008). Relational empathy aims to create a safe trusting space to explore a patient's emotions, gain deeper insights and promote helping behaviour in response to the patient's needs.

BENEFITS OF EMPATHY

Empathy is a way of seeing the world from the point of view of the patient and disadvantaged members of society. Empathy is involved in perspective-taking capabilities that enable doctors to see problems that they might otherwise ignore as moral problems (Maxwell 2008). Relational empathy is person-focused not condition-focused, i.e. it relates to an individual in a particular situation. An empathic relationship confers a number of benefits, including;

Improved Health Outcomes

Emotionally engaged doctors communicate more effectively with patients, decrease patient pain, anxiety and improve their coping strategies, leading to greater therapeutic efficacy and improved patient outcomes (Beck et al. 2002; Derksen et al. 2013; Hegazi and Wilson 2013; Howick et al. 2018; Rietveld and Prins 1998). There is evidence that empathy improves therapeutic effectiveness in other ways; improved immune function, shorter post-operative stay in hospital, fewer asthma episodes, stronger placebo response and even shorter duration of colds (Halpern 2014; Rakel et al. 2009).

Empathy is also associated with greater patient adherence to therapy and so better clinical outcomes (Price et al. 2006; Roter et al. 1998). Empathic understanding is needed not only to understand the patient's illness or emotional reactions but also to understand what is at stake for the patient and to diagnose and treat the patient adequately, to avoid acting against their will and as a core element of informed consent (Pedersen 2010).

Building Trust

The patient-doctor relationship depends on trust in a therapeutic alliance. Qualities in the doctor which foster a good relationship with a patient include empathy and warmth, openness, tolerance and positive regard (Ballatt and Campling 2011). Perhaps the best-understood pathway by which empathy improves health outcomes is the relationship between a patient's perception of the doctor's concern and trust (Halpern 2012; Roter et al. 1998; Roter et al. 1997). It seems that it is not simply the friendliness of the doctor that is the most important factor in engendering trust, but the patient's sense that the doctor is concerned about them and will act in their best interests (Mallia 2013; Roter et al. 1998). Low physician rapport is correlated with a lack of trust as well as increased patient complaints and more malpractice claims (Hickson and Entman 2008).

Concern and Altruism

Batson emphasises just how important protective feelings of concern for the patient in their particular situation are in clinical empathy (Batson et al. 2007). Empathy is also a key element of medical professionalism because it engenders altruism, which gives a higher priority to the patient's interests over those of the doctor (Batson et al. 1991). Halpern hypothesises that patients are most concerned about receiving attentive care. Patients may want their doctors to demonstrate concern because this shows them their doctor has a belief that their suffering is real and takes their needs to be important (Halpern 2012). Conversely, people recovering from psychological trauma describe how an emotionally neutral listener makes them feel insignificant (Halpern 2001).

Patient Satisfaction

Evidence from patients indicates that they want to be seen beyond the manifestations of their illness and to be treated as individuals not just as a list of problems (Ballatt and Campling 2011). Empathic doctors have a sense of shared humanity with patients and their families. Patients express greater satisfaction with doctors who show empathy (Kim et al. 2004; Williams et al. 1998). Research shows that patients want to sense that their doctor is attuned to them before disclosing their deepest concerns (Finset 2010; Suchman et al. 1997). Before patients disclose intimate or emotional issues they often give the doctor non-verbal cues, if the doctor ignores these cues patients may not disclose their real concerns. However, if a doctor is empathic and emotional connection occurs, patients more likely to reveal their real concerns. A better-informed doctor is more likely to make a correct diagnosis and to initiate more appropriate treatment (Halpern 2014).

Enhancing Patient Autonomy

In situations of sickness and suffering, patients may sustain a loss in their autonomy. To exercise autonomy requires being able to see that life is worth continuing and that there is a sense of oneself as an effective agent (Halpern 2001). Suffering often involves a feeling of a loss of self together with feelings of hopelessness and helplessness (Chochinov 2007). Empathic relationships lead to greater patient empowerment, helping patients to recover their autonomy and to imagine a worthwhile future (Bikker et al. 2005; Howie et al. 1999; MacPherson et al. 2003; Price et al. 2006). Once given time and space, a patient may be able to reflect on her emotional responses and perceive a broader view of the reality of her illness regaining a feeling of their true potential (Halpern 2001; Mallia 2013).

A Patient-Orientated Perspective

Empathy provides us with an experiential access to other minds, an ability which can improve with familiarity and practice. However, there are limits to empathy, our understanding of others relies on additional resources. For instance, if we want to understand the reasons why someone is feeling as they do or why they are acting in a certain way we need to consider a wider social and cultural context than can be supplied by empathy alone (Stueber 2006). Halpern suggests that doctors need to be genuinely curious to learn more of the patient's experience (Halpern 2001). She cautions doctors to be careful to avoid taking a self-orientated perspective of the patient when the patient has a similar medical problem or loss that the doctor has experienced themselves. It is easy for the doctor to assume that she knows how the patient is feeling but she must take care to explore the patient's perspective of the situation (Halpern 2012). Clinical curiosity can help to prevent doctors from being naively sympathetic, taking an initial emotional resonance at face value or projecting their own concerns on the patient. Inviting patients to let you know what they are feeling and checking with them that your interpretation is correct are important ways of building trust. Halpern sees empathy as a form of engaged curiosity which goes beyond surface emotions and seeks to understand the patient's whole range of emotions in their particular social setting (Halpern 2014).

A Trusting Patient-Doctor Relationship

An empathic relationship can nurture a sense of safety even in the most uncertain circumstance. Ballatt describes a cycle where attentiveness and kindness enable attunement and generate empathy, while anxiety is reduced (Ballatt and Campling 2011). The resulting trust leads to a better patient-doctor relationship, leading on to improved communication, understanding and patient outcomes. This cycle of empathy and trust has a reinforcing effect so as the relationship continues trust deepens (Ballatt and Campling 2011).

Empathy-Based Ethics

Empathy-based ethics, a fresh relational approach to identify and explore medical ethical dilemmas, is discussed in detail in Chapter 7. Empathy is not just necessary for effective medical practice but it is almost inconceivable for a skilled doctor to lack empathy. Maxwell goes further in extending this general role of empathy to argue that empathy is a capacity which is basic to moral functioning (Maxwell and Racine 2010). Hilfiker argues that a fundamental goal of teaching ethics in medicine should be to foster empathy since empathising is central to perceiving moral problems (Hilfiker 2001). Empathy is a way of seeing the world from the point of view of the patient and disadvantaged members of society. Empathy is involved in perspective-taking capabilities that enable students and doctors to see problems that they might otherwise ignore as moral problems (Maxwell 2008). Empathy can also act as a morally motivating force as the doctor sees things from the patient's point of view. Callahan suggests that it is through emotional and imaginative involvement with others that people come to be concerned about moral problems (Callahan 1980). Recognising a patient's problems and caring about them is what motivates doctors to do their best to help.

Empathy Protects Against Burnout

Low physician empathy is associated with burnout which is linked to lower job satisfaction, leaving medicine, increased substance abuse and suicide (Shanafelt et al. 2005). On the other hand if the doctor is reflective and is curious as to why he/she has negative feelings about a patient or themselves, they may be protected from burnout or compassion fatigue

(Halpern 2014; Sturzu et al. 2019). Using their clinical curiosity, they can reflect on what negative feelings tell them about the patient, and in so doing learn to focus less on their own anxiety and instead concentrate on the patient's feelings (Halpern 2014).

CONCLUSION

Empathy is important in society, in human relationships and ethics. In clinical practice, empathy leads to increased patient and staff satisfaction. Empathy has a role in improving diagnostic accuracy and leads to improved health outcomes for patients. Empathy plays a central role in medical professionalism, the patient-doctor relationship and the development of trust. Empathic doctors suffer less burnout and compassion fatigue and have greater job satisfaction. Respecting a patient's dignity involves relational empathy in seeing the world from their point of view and communicating to the patient that they matter. Empathy is at the core of a new ethical approach: empathy-based ethics.

REFERENCES

Ballatt, J., & Campling, P. (2011). *Intelligent kindness*. London: RCPsych Publications.

Batson, C. D., Batson, J. G., Slingsby, J. K., Harrell, K. L., Peekna, H. M., & Todd, R. M. (1991). Empathic joy and the empathy-altruism hypothesis. *Journal of Personality and Social Psychology, 61*(3), 413–426.

Batson, C. D., Eklund, J. H., Chermok, V. L., Hoyt, J. L., & Ortiz, B. G. (2007). An additional antecedent of empathic concern: Valuing the welfare of the person in need. *Journal of Personality and Social Psychology, 93*(1), 65.

Beck, R. S., Daughtridge, R., & Sloane, P. D. (2002). Physician-patient communication in the primary care office: A systematic review. *The Journal of the American Board of Family Practice, 15*(1), 25–38.

Bikker, A. P., Mercer, S. W., & Reilly, D. (2005). A pilot prospective study on the consultation and relational empathy, patient enablement, and health changes over 12 months in patients going to the Glasgow Homoeopathic Hospital. *Journal of Alternative and Complementary Medicine, 11*(4): 591–600.

Callahan, D. (1980). Goals in the teaching of ethics. In *Ethics teaching in higher education* (pp. 61–80). New York: Springer.

Chochinov, H. (2007). Dignity and the essence of medicine: The A, B, C, and D of dignity conserving care. *BMJ, 335*, 184–187.

Derksen, F., Bensing, J., & Lagro-Janssen, A. (2013). Effectiveness of empathy in general practice: A systematic review. *British Journal General Practice, 63*(606), 76–84.

Finset, A. (2010). Emotions, narrative and empathy in clinical communication. *International Journal of Integrated Care, 10*(Supplement), e020.

Halpern, J. (2001). *From detached concern to empathy: Humanizing medical practice.* Oxford: Oxford University Press.

Halpern, J. (2012). Gathering the patient's story and clinical empathy. *The Permanente Journal, 16, 1.*

Halpern, J. (2014). From idealized clinical empathy to empathic communication in medical care. *Medicine, Health Care and Philosophy, 17*(2), 301–311.

Hegazi, I., & Wilson, I. (2013). Maintaining empathy in medical school: It is possible. *Medical Teacher, 35*(12), 1002–1008.

Hickson, G. B., & Entman, S. S. (2008). Physician practice behavior and litigation risk: Evidence and opportunity. *Clinical Obstetrics and Gynecology, 51*(4), 688–699.

Hilfiker, D. (2001). From the victim's point of view. *Journal of Medical Humanities, 22*(4), 255–263.

Howick, J., Moscrop, A., Mebius, A., Fanshawe, T. R., Lewith, G., Bishop, F. L., ... & Aveyard, P. (2018). Effects of empathic and positive communication in healthcare consultations: a systematic review and meta-analysis. *Journal of the Royal Society of Medicine,* 0141076818769477.

Howie, J. G., Heaney, D. J., Maxwell, M., Walker, J. J., Freeman, G. K., & Rai, H. (1999). Quality at general practice consultations: Cross—Sectional survey. *BMJ, 319*(7212), 738–743.

Kim, S. S., Kaplowitz, S., & Johnston, M. V. (2004). The effects of physician empathy on patient satisfaction and compliance. *Evaluation and the Health Professions, 27*(3), 237–251.

Little, P., Everitt, H., Williamson, I., Warner, G., Moore, M., Gould, C., ... & Payne, S. (2001). Preferences of patients for patient centred approach to consultation in primary care: Observational study. *BMJ, 322*(7284), 1–7.

MacPherson, H., Mercer, S. W., Scullion, T., & Thomas, K. J. (2003). Empathy, enablement, and outcome: An exploratory study on acupuncture patients' perceptions. *The Journal of Alternative & Complementary Medicine, 9*(6), 869–876.

Mallia, P. (2013). *The nature of the doctor-patient relationship: Health care principles through the phenomenology of relationships with patients.* Dordrecht: Springer.

Maxwell, B. (2008). *Professional ethics education: Studies in compassionate empathy.* New York: Springer.

Maxwell, B., & Racine, E. (2010). Should empathic development be a priority in biomedical ethics teaching? A critical perspective. *Cambridge Quarterly of Healthcare Ethics, 19*(4), 433–445.

Noddings, N. (2013). *Caring: A relational approach to ethics and moral education.* Berkeley, CA: University of California Press.

Pedersen, R. (2010). Empathy development in medical education—A critical review. *Medical Teacher, 32*(7), 593–600.

Price, S., Mercer, S. W., & MacPherson, H. (2006). Practitioner empathy, patient enablement and health outcomes: A prospective study of acupuncture patients. *Patient Education and Counseling, 63*(1), 239–245.

Rakel, D. P., Hoeft, T. J., Barrett, B. P., Chewning, B. A., Craig, B. M., & Niu, M. (2009). Practitioner empathy and the duration of the common cold. *Family Medicine, 41*(7), 494–501.

Rietveld, S., & Prins, P. (1998). The relationship between negative emotions and acute subjective and objective symptoms of childhood asthma. *Psychological Medicine, 28*(02), 407–415.

Roter, D. L., Hall, J. A., Merisca, R., Nordstrom, B., Cretin, D., & Svarstad, B. (1998). Effectiveness of interventions to improve patient compliance: A meta-analysis. *Medical Care, 36*(8), 1138–1161.

Roter, D. L., Stewart, M., Putnam, S. M., Lipkin, M., Stiles, W., & Inui, T. S. (1997). Communication patterns of primary care physicians. *JAMA, 277*(4), 350–356.

Shanafelt, T. D., West, C., Zhao, X., Novotny, P., Kolars, J., Habermann, T., & Sloan, J. (2005). Relationship between increased personal well-being and enhanced empathy among internal medicine residents. *Journal of General Internal Medicine, 20*(7), 559–564.

Stewart, M. (2001). Towards a global definition of patient centred care. *BMJ, 322*(7284), 444–445.

Stueber, K. (2006). *Rediscovering empathy: Agency.* Folk Psychology and the Human Sciences Cambridge Mass: MIT Press.

Sturzu, L., Lala, A., Bisch, M., Guitter, M., Dobre, D., & Schwan, R. (2019). Empathy and burnout—A cross-sectional study among mental healthcare providers in France. *Journal of Medicine and Life, 12*, 21–29.

Suchman, A. L., Markakis, K., Beckman, H. B., & Frankel, R. (1997). A model of empathic communication in the medical interview. *JAMA, 277*(8), 678–682.

Williams, S., Weinman, J., & Dale, J. (1998). Doctor–patient communication and patient satisfaction. *Family Practice, 15*, 480–492.

CHAPTER 7

Empathy-Based Ethics (EBE): A New Approach to Clinical Ethics

Abstract Empathy-based ethics (EBE) is better suited to a humane form of clinical practice than standard judgemental theoretical bioethical approaches. In establishing the need for a fresh empathy-based approach, current models of medical ethics are briefly reviewed: deontology and utilitarianism. The limitations of the four-principle approach, autonomy (self-determination), beneficence (doing good), non-maleficence (do not harm) and justice (being fair), are debated. Virtue ethics and care ethics are outlined and their relevance to the empathy-based approach discussed. The empathy-based approach is described and discussed. At its core is relational empathy as manifest in the patient-doctor relationship. Moral sensitivity and reflection combine in moral judgement, drive motivation, to result in action to help the patient. A reflection on the limitations of an empathy-based approach, including bias, helps to strengthen the argument for adopting this form of clinical ethics.

Keywords Empathy-based ethics · Deontology · Utilitarianism · Four-principle approach · Limitations of empathy

© The Author(s), under exclusive license to Springer Nature
Switzerland AG 2020
D. I. Jeffrey, *Empathy-Based Ethics*,
https://doi.org/10.1007/978-3-030-64804-6_7

73

INTRODUCTION

Ethics is concerned with how to act, how to live or what kind of person to be (Kagan 1998). Medical ethics concerns the moral values, attitudes, behaviour and judgement of doctors when faced with moral dilemmas in their practice. Empathy is a unique way in which doctors connect emotionally with patients to understand what is at stake for them and to help identify and guide ethical judgement. Empathy depends upon relationship, in this case that between a patient and a doctor (Maibom 2014). As empathy is intrinsic to medical ethics, this chapter argues for a fresh approach, empathy-based ethics (EBE), which is better suited to a humane form of clinical practice than standard judgemental theoretical bioethical approaches. Considering ethical issues through an 'empathy lens' is a key part of redressing the biomedical-psychosocial imbalance and so humanising medicine. Empathy, at the centre of moral life, acknowledges that every individual is of equal worth (Garrett 2014).

The relational view of empathy adopted in this book proposes that a doctor takes the subjective perspectives, cognitive and affective of the patient, reflects on their state of mind and imagines how things are (were, or will be) for that individual. The doctor imagines how she would think and feel if she was in the patient's situation and with this empathic concern is motivated to assist the patient (Garrett 2014). In arguing for an empathic approach to clinical ethics to meet the demand for more humane care, current models of medical ethics are briefly reviewed and the need for empathy-based ethics (EBE) explored.

Moral aspects of empathy are relatively little researched in the medical literature. The development of empathy-based ethics is traced from the time of Enlightenment philosophers, Hume and Smith, to the present day. The contribution of empathy to ethics and morality is described with a discussion of the limitations of empathy-based ethics. Moral aspects of empathy are explored in theoretical terms in this chapter and followed in Chapter 8, by examples of empathy-based ethics in clinical practice.

MEDICAL ETHICS

Historically medical ethics, was concerned with the duties and responsibilities of a doctor, enshrined in codes dating from the Hippocratic oath (460–370 BC) (Miles 2005). Hippocrates claimed that a love of humanity was integral to the art of medicine, emphasising the enduring centrality of empathy in the patient-doctor relationship (Weir et al. 2015). Thomas Percival published 'Medical Ethics' in 1803, a code of principles of conduct for doctors and their relationship with society (Marcum 2008).The American Medical Association produced a code of ethics in 1847 which stressed scientific medical knowledge rather than the character of a physician (Marcum 2008).

Medical ethics developed as 'bioethics' in the 1960s, initially directed at a perceived dehumanisation of medicine by an overemphasis of technical and scientific aspects. The initial aim was to instil human values into medicine and nursing through education which included the humanities (Pellegrino 1999). However, in the 1970s technical advances in medicine such as organ transplantation, human experimentation and genetic engineering revealed a need for systematic philosophical analysis in resolving ethical dilemmas. Beauchamp and Childress defined a four-principle approach to bioethics to act an ethical guide to medical decision-making (Beauchamp and Childress 2013). More recently global issues have widened the scope of bioethics to include psychosocial, economic legal and religious issues. Pellegrino commenting on the development of bioethics concluded, "the original hoped-for humanisation of medical education and practice remains an elusive ideal" (Pellegrino 1999). Since the main philosophical approaches adopted in medical ethics have failed to achieve the humanisation of medical practice, this chapter will explore reasons for this deficiency and argue for an empathy-based approach.

ETHICAL FRAMEWORKS

Ethical frameworks can assist doctors and patients in their decision-making. The following frameworks are commonly used in current clinical practice.

Deontology

Deontology is a duty-based approach to ethics advocated by Kant (1724–1804), who believed that it was imperative to treat people as individuals of equal moral worth and never as a means to an end (Jeffrey 2006; Scruton 2001). Doctors have special obligations, or duties, to care for patients. Deontology is action-based, each action is subject to moral scrutiny and the intentions of a doctor are morally relevant. Doctors adopting a Kantian approach feel more comfortable in doing the best for the individual patient in front of them rather than considering the needs of the wider community. For Kant, morality is not about consequences or maximising happiness but rather about respecting people and considering the moral intentions of any action (Sandel 2009).

Pure practical reason is Kant's main principle, we are rational beings capable of choosing freely and acting autonomously (Kant 1998). In Kantian thought, to be autonomous is to be governed by a law I give myself, introducing a caveat of responsibility. Acting autonomously, I do not simply do as I wish but instead, step back from my own interests and reflect on a proposed course of action as a person with pure practical reason (Sandel 2009).

Kant described a 'categorical imperative' sometimes call universalisability; "act only on that maxim whereby you can at the same time will that it should become a universal law" (Kant 1998; Sandel 2009). This test is a moral check to see if an action I am about to undertake puts my interests above everyone else's (Sandel 2009).It is also the basis of the 'golden rule' that we should do as we would be done by (Scruton 2001). For Kant, respecting human dignity means treating people as ends in themselves.

Deontology is an absolute moral theory in setting out clear moral rules which are binding in all cultures, e.g. do not kill (Marcum 2008). Doing the right thing is to perform one's duty by following an absolute rule. Kant's use of pure practical reason in making moral judgements ignores emotions, its cold rational approach does not seem to fit with the complexity of clinical practice nor with the project of humanising medical care. Patients do not want doctors to view them simply as professional duties but as unique individuals for whom the doctor has some genuine feeling (Marcum 2008; Tong 2007). When moral absolutes conflict, there is no clear way of choosing between them, for example, a request from an autonomous patient for euthanasia. The question arises, how far should an absolute rule be followed? For instance, the rule to tell the truth would prohibit lying under any circumstance, however harmful the consequences.

Utilitarianism

Utilitarianism claims that the happiness, or utility, for the greatest number is the greatest moral good. (Marcum 2008) In this theory, it is the consequence of an action which is of moral concern. Utilitarianism was proposed by JS Mill 1806–1873 and J Bentham (1748–1832), claiming that whatever maximises utility is morally right. JS Mill believed that people should be free to do whatever they want, provided that they do no harm to others (Sandel 2009).Utilitarian theory may appeal to politicians, healthcare managers and public health doctors seeking primarily to benefit the greatest number of people (Jeffrey 2006).

The first problem encountered in utilitarianism is how one can define happiness or utility. It is also difficult to calculate optimal utility as unforeseen or unintended consequences may affect the outcome of any action. There is a risk that in attempting to maximise utility for the greatest number, an important vulnerable minority may be overlooked. For instance, in a viral pandemic, resources may be focused on infected patients while neglecting the needs of those with other diseases. In contrast, empathy-based ethics is most concerned with the rights of vulnerable patients who deserve respect, each individual is of equal moral value.

The question arises does the end justify the means? Utilitarian justify an act (the means) in terms of its consequence (end), seeming to conflict with a humane form of medical practice. There have been notorious examples of unethical human experimentation, such as the infamous Tuskegee study (1932–1972) on the natural history of syphilis. In this study, 400 African Americans with syphilis were left untreated despite antibiotics becoming available, causing a public outcry (Marcum 2008).

Yet another difficulty with Utilitarian theory is deriving moral theory from people's desires. Just because something gives a person pleasure does not necessarily make it morally right (Marcum 2008). Morality cannot be based on simply the interests, wants and desires that people have at any one point in time, variable factors which should not form the basis of universal moral principles (Sandel 2009).

Principlism

Western medical practice has largely adopted the four-principle approach to thinking about ethical dilemmas. Developed by Beauchamp and Childress they include (Beauchamp and Childress 2013);

Autonomy (self-determination)
Beneficence (doing good)

Non-maleficence (do not harm)
Justice (being fair)

Autonomy

Autonomy is the capacity to think, decide and act on the basis of such thought and decision, freely and independently (Gillon 1985). In expressing autonomy, an individual shapes and gives meaning to their life. Autonomy may be respected in many ways; telling the truth, preserving confidentiality and obtaining informed consent.

Ethical dilemmas may occur in the conflict between patient autonomy and medical power. For example, when a patient with breast cancer refuses chemotherapy, there may be a conflict between a doctor's duty of beneficence and respecting her autonomy. Any medical intervention carries a risk of paternalism and a potential threat to the patient's autonomy. A requirement for informed consent protects the patient's autonomy from such paternalism (Jeffrey 2006). There are differing interpretations of autonomy, those stressing independence rather than responsibility for others may generate selfish choices from such an impaired interpretation of autonomy (Marcum 2008).

Beneficence

This principle emphasises the moral importance of doing good to patients (Hope 2004). Medical practice is grounded in the principle of beneficence, patients trust that the doctor will act in their best interests (Mallia 2013).This seems clear at first glance, but the question arises, who should be the judge of what is best for the patent? Doctors try to act in the patient's best interests but judging these is often complicated and uncertain. It should also be remembered that paternalism is often driven by a doctor's unchecked beneficence.

Non-maleficence

'Do no harm' is a Hippocratic maxim familiar to every medical student and doctor. However, this principle often is in conflict with beneficence. For example, a patient with breast cancer may undergo mutilating surgery in the hope of cure. Striking a balance between the risks and benefits of treatments is often difficult.

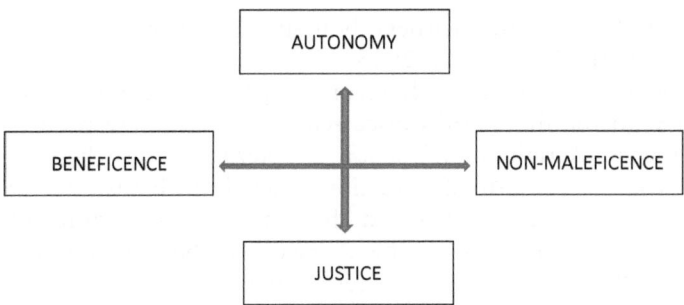

Fig. 7.1   The four principles

Justice
Distributive justice is concerned that patients in similar situations should
have the same access to health care (Hope 2004). Additionally, healthcare
resources should be distributed fairly between different groups of patients.
Issues of autonomy may clash with justice, for example, when a patient
is denied treatment with an expensive new experimental drug to preserve
proven resources for other patients.

Although the four principles assist in clarifying thinking, the principles
often clash when applied to individual clinical dilemmas, when it may be
difficult to decide which principle should have priority. Principlism is not
an algorithm for resolving ethical dilemmas as there is no systematic way
of dealing with conflicts between them (Fig. 7.1).

Virtue Ethics

Virtue ethics is an ethical framework that emphasises the virtues or
moral character rather than rules or consequences (Hursthouse 1999).
There is renewed interest in medical ethics in classic virtue theory origi-
nally described by Aristotle (Arthur et al. 2015). Pellegrino recommends
retaining the four principles but supplementing them with insights from
other ethical theories such as virtue ethics (Pellegrino 1994). Virtue
theory is concerned with the moral integrity and character of the doctor
rather than with moral rules or principles. Aristotle's concept of aspiring
to practical wisdom *(phronesis)* is central to virtue ethics. Aristotle main-
tained that leading a virtuous life was *eudaimonia*, to be in a state of
flourishing. Recent research on the virtues of a good doctor listed six

important characteristics: fairness, honesty, judgement, kindness, leadership, teamwork (Arthur et al. 2015).

Although virtue ethics would seem to support more humane medicine, compared to the frameworks discussed earlier, there are problems with virtue theory. A right moral action is determined by what a virtuous person would do in a similar situation. Therefore what is good in a situation must be identified first and there may be many different goods to consider as well as taking the character of the doctor into account (Marcum 2008).Virtue theory shares another challenge with principlism, determining the precedence of the various virtues.

Care Ethics

Care ethics emerged in 1988 as part of second-wave feminisim (Gilligan 1982; Noddings 1984). Instead of principles or rules, care ethics takes 'care' as its core (van Dijke et al. 2019). Caring involves a mutual relationship of seeing and responding to need (Gilligan 1982). It involves moral attention, understanding and mutual trust. Care ethics is a relational branch of ethics, it places a high value on emotions and takes account of context. It has a political dimension in its awareness of the power dimensions implicated in care (van Dijke et al. 2019). Care ethicists view humans as inherently vulnerable and mutually dependent, stressing that we all depend on care during some stage of our lives (van Dijke et al. 2019). Some claim that to be human means being in caring relationships with other people (van Dijke et al. 2019).

Care ethics is sceptical of universal principles since they cannot do justice to the richness and complexity of a particular moral situation, to the relationship between people and to individual values and needs. Care ethics pays attention to insights emerging from attentive relationships and from a sensitivity to context, in its relational humane approach it shares many aspects of empathy-based ethics. Slote argues that empathy should form the foundation of care ethics (Slote 2007). Empathy is thought to be foundational because it makes doctors care for patients. Empathy-based ethics is a development of the ideas embodied in care ethics and better suited to medical practice.

EMPATHY-BASED ETHICS

Background

Empathy-based ethics is essentially relational, at its heart is the patient-doctor relationship. Empathy-based ethics has its roots in the Scottish Enlightenment. David Hume (1711–1776) described a concept of sympathy to explain phenomena such as sharing of emotions and the formation of moral responses (Hume 1739/1978). Hume described sympathy as fellow feeling, characterising it as a natural and automatic process which could be equated today with emotional resonance or sympathy. Hume thought moral judgements must be based in sympathy but also from a common point of view (Hume 1739/1978). Hume also noted that we feel more for those close to us in affection, time and place, pointing to a tendency to bias (Hume 1739/1978). Adam Smith (1723–1790) added imaginative perspective-taking to Hume's concept of sympathy to form a 'sympathy' which is similar to our concept of empathy today (Smith (1759/1976)). Smith also described an ideal observer of the target situation, unaffected by bias (Smith (1759/1976)).

Kant's rationalist moral judgements, grounded in pure practical reason have become less fashionable (Maibon 2014). There is now some scepticism about the predominant role of reason in moral judgement and the neglect of emotions. In the search for a more humane form of ethics Hume and Smith's views have again become more relevant (Coplan and Goldie 2011). One of the fascinations of philosophy is how often we return to ideas from the past and apply them to today's dilemmas. Empathy-based ethics (EBE) is a fresh approach to clinical ethics, drawing on care ethics and the virtues, centred on the patient-doctor relationship and extending to promote a humane form of medical practice.

THE MORALITY OF EMPATHY

Relational empathy, conceptualised in broad terms can act as a moral compass as it obliges doctors to care for patients and to listen to their concerns (Maibom 2014). Empathy plays important moral roles, in an orientating the doctor towards the patient and in moral judgement (Maibon 2014). R.M. Hare claimed that to behave in a truly moral way we have to "know what it is like" for [the other person] (Hare 1981). Others have argued that empathy is central to morality (Kauppinen 2013). While Oxley accepts that empathy is essential for a moral life, she cautions that it is not the sole basis of ethics, since empathy does not always lead to moral action (Oxley 2011).

In valuing difference, empathy has the power to be a 'social glue' and broaden our horizons (Maibom 2017). Hoffman suggests that empathy sparks concern for others, making social life possible (Hoffman 2000). Broad relational empathy which relates to sympathy, kindness, generosity and humility is a different construct from the narrow cognitive empathy, or detached concern, prevalent in medical practice today.

The empathy-based ethics approach incorporates and develops Rest's psychological moral model (Rest 1986) (Fig. 7.2).

Moral Sensitivity

Moral sensitivity involves perceiving a situation as presenting a moral problem and imagining the effects of different courses of action on the patient's welfare (Rest 1986). Empathy brings new information to our attention, as it one of the few ways we have of connecting with another's emotions and point of view (Oxley 2011).Empathy can tell us what is at stake for others and alert us to a call for an ethical response (van Dijke et al. 2019). A doctor entertains different beliefs, adopting a different view of the world to recreate the patient's perspective.

Moral Imagination

Empathy is a perceptive capacity that allows doctors to see problems they might otherwise ignore as ethical problems and moves them to act to help the patient (Hilfiker 2001). Callahan claims that moral imagination attunes the doctor to threats to the well-being of the patient and motivates her to solve the ethical problem. A doctor starts thinking about the world from the patient's perspective, imagining reasons for possible actions and thoughts. Empathy is a form of moral imagination which can help doctors to understand or predict the impact of medical interventions on others (van Dijke et al. 2019).

Emotions

Imagining being in the patient's situation and acquiring a congruent emotion is at the heart of empathy (Oxley 2011). Empathy involves both

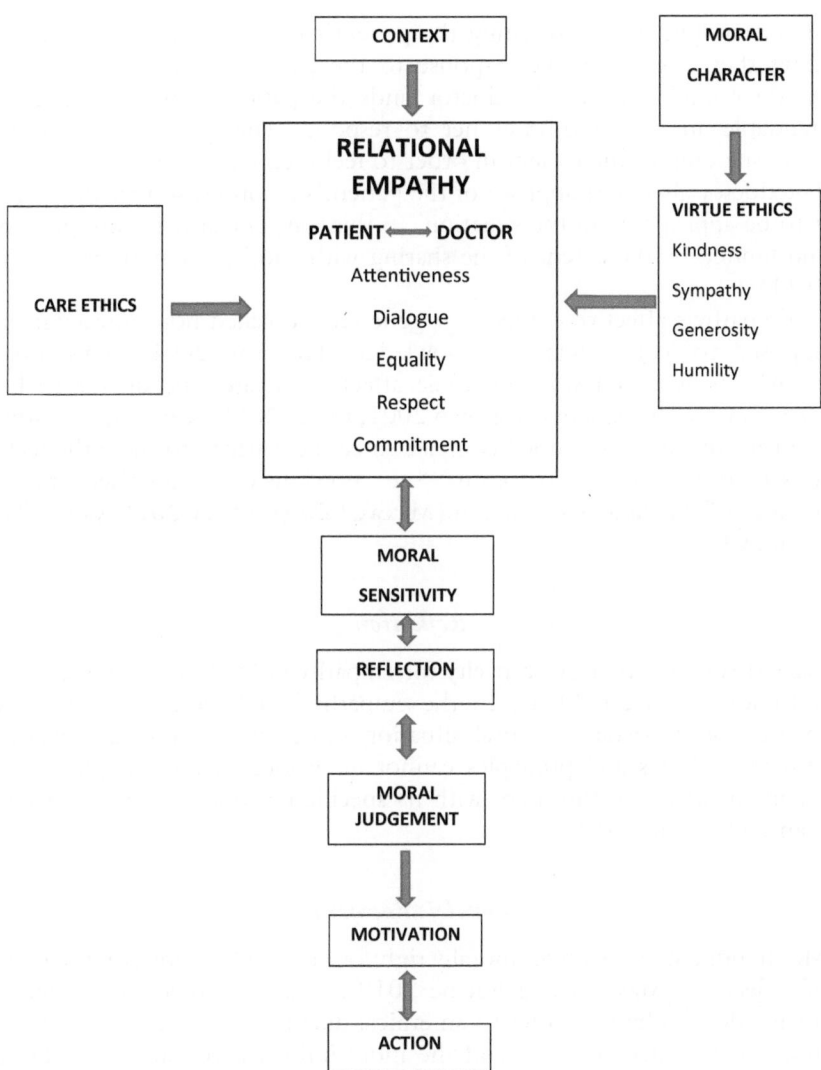

Fig. 7.2 An empathy-based ethics approach

understanding and appreciating the patient's feelings and not just imagining them. An empathic response to the patient's emotions depends on their intelligibility. The doctor finds the patient's emotions understandable and this motivates her to respond. The doctor needs some understanding of the patient in order to feel their emotions and respond. The doctor also must approve of the patient's emotions so that they take it to be appropriate in the situation. In this way, empathy is both guided and limited by the extent of the sharing with another's emotions (Oxley 2011).

Empathy's affective component generates so-called hot knowledge as opposed to 'cool', detached knowledge (Hoffman 2001). This 'hot' knowledge, charged with empathic affect, motivates the doctor to be responsive to the patient (Hoffman 2001; Oxley 2011). Genuine empathy can thus function as a moral compass since the capacity to share the feelings of others allows doctors to "see" previously unrecognised ethical features of the patient's situation (Maxwell 2008; Oxley 2011; van Dijke et al. 2019).

Reflection

Garrett suggests that our capacity for empathy needs to be "infused with reflection" (Garrett 2014). In the empathy-based model, reflection is focused on a particular moral situation rather than applying universal principles. Rules and principles cannot do justice to the complexity of a patient-doctor relationship, with its specific personal values and needs (van Dijke et al. 2019).

Moral Judgements

Moral judgement identifies morally right or preferable actions on the basis of reflection (Maxwell and Racine 2010). It is the process by which a doctor decides how to react to an ethical dilemma. Doctors aim to work in a patient's best interests and the more informed the doctor is about the patient and their situation the better their judgement is likely to be (Garrett 2014). A doctor can only judge what is best for a patient by having access to their subjective perspectives through empathy. Garrett summarises; "empathy is a doorway to understanding what is best for anyone" (Garrett 2014). Empathic deliberation involves thinking about the patient's relevant feelings and desires and the way in which they perceive their lives (Oxley 2011). Empathic deliberation matures to moral empathic deliberation when guided by insights from care ethics and the virtues. It involves a doctor feeling the patient's emotions and appreciating their situation in ways that enable them to be more sensitive to the moral values at stake (Oxley 2011). A doctor bases their interpretation of the patient's actions and emotions on the knowledge gained in the earlier parts of the consultation. Empathy can lead to moral concern or even outrage and so influence moral judgement (Maibom 2014).

Empathy can serve as a criterion whether an action is morally right, reflecting Hume and Smith's ideas that an action is morally good when based on broadly based empathic concern. Concern for the well-being of others is an essential element of ordinary moral judgement. Rawls suggests that the presence of an ideal observer would reduce bias. This process requires reflective judgement on another's feelings situation reasons and desires, not simply the discovery of their preferences, so utilising empathy in his moral decision-making process (Rawls 2009).

After the process of moral reflection the doctor then uses their own virtues, insights from care ethics, experience and wisdom to make a moral judgement (Oxley 2011). Empathy can generate new insights and beliefs about others, expanding our knowledge and transforming existing beliefs. Given empathy's tendency to bias, a virtuous type of empathy, without prejudice, has been described as mature empathy (Oxley 2011).

Motivation

Moral motivation is a drive to derive the best possible solution to moral problems (Callahan 1980). Humans have innate empathic abilities, making them relational and altruistic beings (Batson 2011b; de Waal 2012). Darwin noted the evolutionary advantage conferred by acting for the good of the group (Darwin 2013). Relational empathy has a strong affective component which includes a caring involvement in the patient's suffering and a sense of shared humanity (Maxwell and Racine 2010). Empathy involves understanding the other's perspectives and feeling their emotions, putting their concerns and needs ahead of one's own (Oxley 2011). Batson defines altruism as, 'a motivational state with the ultimate goal of increasing another's welfare' (Batson 2014). Acting altruistically depends upon taking an other-oriented perspective which generates appropriate empathic concern. Empathy, in responding to suffering, promotes altruism and helping behaviours (Batson et al.

2009; Garden 2009). Altruism is based on helping the patient but carries a risk of paternalism, a risk that may be reduced by a requirement for the patient's informed consent.

Action

Kaplan describes empathy that does not result in helping behaviour as 'empty empathy' (Kaplan 2011). Actions are morally good when based on fully developed empathic concern (Slote 2007; van Dijke et al. 2019). Care ethics suggest that the more we empathise the greater our moral obligation, as our moral obligations are derived from empathy (Slote 2007).

LIMITATION OF EMPATHY-BASED ETHICS

Prinz argues that empathy is not necessary for moral judgement, motivation or moral development (Prinz 2011a, 2011b). Kant, as a rationalist, argued strongly for moral judgements to be grounded in pure practical reason (Kant 1998).

Examining the limitations of the empathy-based ethical approach helps to develop new insights which may refine the model. The new approach draws on care ethics and the virtues to create a relational empathy-based ethics which can benefit both the patient and doctor.

Definitions

People use the word empathy to mean different things which leads to disagreement about the value of the concept (Garrett 2014). The different ways of conceptualising empathy make it difficult to unravel some of the arguments surrounding the concept. Clarifying this confusion by adopting a broad relational view of empathy is a first step towards more humane care (Jeffrey 2016).

Macnaughton described empathy as 'dangerous', warning of "the way in which medicine can highjack complex ideas, confining them and defining them in its own terms and changing their meaning and impact". She favours a cognitive model of empathy, arguing that in clinical practice, "one person meets the other not as a fellow being but as a type of a person: as 'doctor or patient'" (Macnaughton 2009). Defining empathy narrowly as a cognitive construct further distances doctor and patient leading to critiques against empathy as a foundation for a relational form of ethics (van Dijke et al. 2019). However, as empathy is essentially relational, a doctor should regard a patient as a fellow human being, not solely as an object of clinical interest.

Bloom, in his book '*Against Empathy*', defined empathy in purely affective terms, then asserted that this narrowly defined empathy created a bias against patients. Instead, he proposed a form of 'rational compassion', which seemed similar to the broad form of empathy for which I have argued in this book (Bloom 2016). Prinz also defines empathy in largely emotional terms in his critique which concludes that empathy is not ideally suited as a basis of morality (Prinz 2011b). Critics of empathy tend to equate it with identification, but empathy, unlike identification, crucially retains a sense of a psychological boundary between the self and the other (Bondi 2003; Macnaughton 2009; Watson and Greenburg 2011).

Authors have suggested that emotional connection with the patient was unnecessary, politeness was sufficient to meet the patient's needs. They justified this claim by suggesting that objectivity protected the doctor and that distancing from the patient was therefore essential in medical practice (Smajdor et al. 2011). However, rather than enforcing a choice between objectivity or connection with a patient, they conceded that they might co-exist by a switching between modes depending on the clinical context.

Bias

Some authors claim empathy is biased and may be distorted by prejudices (Maibom 2014; Noddings 2013). There are different kinds of potential empathy bias (van Dijke et al. 2019). Familiarity bias occurs as we tend to empathise with those close to us (Hoffman 2001). There is support from psychology and neuroscience research that empathy is easier amongst friends rather than strangers (Hoffman 2001; Meyer et al. 2013). There is also a risk that we tend to empathise with those whose feelings are congruent with our own. This limitation is reduced in relational empathy since it aims to connect with the other person at a deeper level and values difference (Jeffrey 2017). It is easier to empathise with those who are physically present than with those who are absent, a potential for a "here and now" bias (Hoffman 2014). Hoffman suggests that countering this bias is possible by deliberately taking the perspective of those who are not present (Hoffman 2014).

Kauppinen discusses emotion regulation in moral judgement by suggesting down-regulating empathy with nearest and dearest and up-regulating empathy for people who are different or distant (Kauppinen 2014). Adopting Rawls' Veil of Ignorance, he suggests deliberating from the perspective of a sympathetic impartial spectator (Kauppinen 2014; Rawls 2009). Hume suggested a perspective from 'the common point of view' to guide moral judgements (Hume 1739/1978).The crucial question is not whether we are more empathic to those who are closer to us but whether we have the potential to be equally empathic to people removed from us in time or space (Garrett 2014). We need to see all others as human beings like ourselves, having equal moral worth and so extend our capacity for empathy. Empathic bias might occasionally function as a filtering mechanism to focus empathic attention, rendering it manageable, since understanding everyone's point of view and feeling everyone's pain is clearly impractical (Maxwell 2008).

Stereotyping and prejudice are possible results of bias but relational empathy aims to be non-judgemental. However, any empathy bias can be corrected by incorporating lessons from care ethics and the virtues. Despite the fact that people empathise most strongly with those they identify with on the basis of race, culture belief or values, empathy can nevertheless transform people and thus transform their perception of others (Oxley 2011). Empathy can be the antidote to prejudice by enabling doctors to see what is important to patients in seeing things from their point of view (Oxley 2011).

Respect for the patient's dignity is another antidote to any possible bias (Chochinov 2007; Meyers 1994). Empathic dialogue reduces the possibility of prejudice, by seeing others as they see themselves, not as our culture has defined them (Oxley 2011). Mature or virtuous empathy involves being perceptive to the other's complex moral and social situation to grasp who they are as a person (Oxley 2011). Respect for the other as a human being is a prerequisite for mature empathy. One must be able to see and feel how another person's life and perspectives are valuable (Oxley 2011). It requires both intellectual and emotional openness towards others especially those who are radically different from oneself.

Empathic Accuracy

Some ethicists have concerns about the problem of empathic accuracy, doubting if it is possible to acquire accurate knowledge of others using empathy (Tronto 1993). Macnaughton claimed that a full experience of mutuality or understanding of another person was not possible (Macnaughton 2009). It is possible that well-intended actions based on inaccurate information could lead to paternalism and end in harm (van Dijke et al. 2019). The counter-argument is that although a full understanding of another person may not be possible, patients should still be treated respectfully in the clinical encounter (Halpern 2001).

These objections emphasise the need for reflection, checking with the patient that empathy has led to a sharing of accurate knowledge. Accuracy of empathic imagination depends also on how much information the doctor has about the patient and the extent to which she aims to genuinely imagine the patient's perspective (Oxley 2011). At a time when personalised continuity of care is uncommon, it becomes less likely that the doctor will know the patient.

Burnout and Personal Distress

While Reiss acknowledged the benefits of empathy in clinical practice both to patients and doctors, she questioned whether empathy must entail an emotional cost to healthcare professionals (Riess 2015). Batson proposed that empathy, shown as appropriate empathetic concern, need not include personal distress (Batson 2011). Personal distress, a result of taking a self-orientated perspective, may cause the doctor to cease empathising and to distance themselves from the patient (Hoffman 2001).

The context of the encounter may also contribute to emotional overload rather than fostering empathetic concern; for instance, if time is short or the workload excessive, emotional distress may follow (Gleichgerrcht and Decety 2013). Empathic doctors require support and an opportunity to share concerns with colleagues (Jeffrey 2014). The evidence suggests that rather than resulting in burnout, relational empathy protects against burnout (Kearney et al. 2009; Sturzu et al. 2019).

CONCLUSION: THE EMPATHY-BASED ETHICS APPROACH

A broad relational view of empathy encompasses the patient and doctor in a caring relationship. Empathy overlaps with concepts of kindness, generosity, sympathy and humility and includes the philosophy of care ethics. Consideration of virtue ethics is relevant to the concept of a good doctor. Within a relationship based on empathy, there is a dialogue involving reflection which includes elements of moral perception, emotions and imagination. Moral judgement involves empathy and takes account of the particular context of the individuals' situation. In a relational model, the patient and doctor work in a partnership in decision-making with a requirement for informed consent, action follows as empathy is a response to suffering.

Examining the critiques of empathy-based ethics, bias and inaccuracy provokes a deeper understanding of the functions of the approach. As Macnaughton suggested, there are limits to empathy, to understand others there is a need to consider a wider social and cultural context than can be supplied by empathy alone (Macnaughton 2009). Halpern proposed that doctors needed to approach this dilemma by being genuinely curious to learn more of the patient's experience (Halpern 2001). She argued that clinical curiosity can help to prevent doctors from being naively sympathetic or projecting their own concerns on the patient. Empathy as a form of engaged curiosity goes beyond surface emotions and seeks to understand the patient's experience, by adopting a phenomenological approach (Halpern 2014; Vagle 2016).

There is a need to embrace a broad view of relational empathy and to emphasise the need for an ethical pause for reflection. Doctors need to be self-aware of the possibility of bias and seek to understand patients not to judge them. The evolution of empathy-based ethics from care ethics is in part a result of addressing these limitations (Freedberg 2007). Empathy-based ethics considers both the patient and the doctor as active participants in the consultation.

Empathy-based ethics has greater relevance to current medical practice than rule-based approaches. It is fundamentally relational, focusing on the patient-doctor relationship and adopting a broad concept of empathy. Relational empathy values cultural differences, broadening our horizons and in the process transforming us (van Dijke et al. 2019). The question arises as to how to embed an empathy-based approach into medical practice, education and research to support good care and prevent physician's personal distress (van Dijke et al. 2019). The next chapter describes how this might occur in practice by analysing three difficult clinical ethical dilemmas.

REFERENCES

Arthur, J., et al. (2015). *Virtuous medical practice*. Jubilee Centre for Character and Virtue: Birmingham.

Batson, C. D., Ahmad, N., & Lishner, D. A. (2009). Empathy and altruism. In C. Snyder & S. Lopez (Eds.), *Oxford handbook of positive psychology* (pp. 417–427). Oxford: Oxford University Press.

Batson, C. (2011). These things called empathy: Eight related but distinct phenomena. In J. Decety & W. Ickes *The social neuroscience of empathy* (pp. 6–15). Cambridge, MA: MIT Press.

Batson, C. D. (2011). *Altruism in humans*. Oxford: Oxford University Press.

Batson, C. D. (2014). Empathy-induced altruism and morality. In H. L. Maibom (Ed.), *Empathy and morality*. Oxford: Oxford University Press.

Beauchamp, T., & Childress, J. (2013). *Principles of biomedical ethics*. New York: Oxford University Press.

Bloom, P. (2016). *Against empathy: The case for rational compassion*. London: The Bodley Head.

Bondi, L. (2003). Empathy and identification: Conceptual resources for feminist fieldwork. *ACME: An international E-journal for critical geographies, 2*(1), 64–76.

Callahan, D. (1980). Goals in the teaching of ethics. *Ethics teaching in higher education* (pp. 61–80). New York: Springer.

Chochinov, H. (2007). Dignity and the essence of medicine: the A, B, C, and D of dignity conserving care. *BMJ, 335,* 184–187.

Coplan, A. & Goldie, P. (Eds.). (2011). *Empathy: Philosophical and psychological perspectives*. Oxford: Oxford University Press.

Darwin, C. (2013). *The descent of man*. London: Wordsworth Editions.

de Waal, F. B. (2012). *The age of empathy: Nature's lessons for a kinder society*. London: Souvenir Press Ltd.

Freedberg, S. (2007). Re-examining empathy: A relational—Femminist point of view. *Social Work, 52,* 251–259.

Garden, R. (2009). Expanding clinical empathy: An activist perspective. *Journal of General Internal Medicine, 24*(1), 122–125.

Garrett, K. R. (2014). At the empathetic center of our moral lives. In H. Maibom (Ed.), *Empathy and morality*. Oxford: Oxford University Press.

Gilligan, C. (1982). *In a different voice: Psychological theory and womens' development*. Cambridge: Harvard University Press.

Gillon, R. (1985). *Philosophical medical ethics*. Chichester: John Wiley & Sons.

Gleichgerrcht, E., & Decety, J. (2013). Empathy in clinical practice: How individual dispositions, gender, and experience moderate empathic concern, burnout, and emotional distress in physicians. *PLoS ONE, 8,* e61526. https://doi.org/10.1371/journal.pone.0061526.

92   D. I. JEFFREY

Halpern, J. (2001). *From detached concern to empathy: Humanizing medical practice*. Oxford: Oxford University Press.

Halpern, J. (2014). From idealized clinical empathy to empathic communication in medical care. *Medicine, Health Care and Philosophy, 17*(2), 301–311.

Hare, R. M. (1981). *Moral thinking*. Oxford: Clarendon.

Hilfiker, D. (2001). From the victim's point of view. *Journal of Medical Humanities, 22*(4), 255–263.

Hoffman, M. L. (2000). *Empathy and moral development: Implications for caring and justice*. Cambridge, MA: Cambridge University Press.

Hoffman, M. L. (2001). *Empathy and moral development: Implications for caring and justice*. Cambridge: Cambridge University Press.

Hoffman, M. L. (2014). Empathy justice and social change. In H. L. Maibon (Ed.), *Empathy and morality*. Oxford: Oxford University Press.

Hope, T. (2004). *Medical ethics: A very short introduction*. Oxford: Oxford University Press.

Hume, D. (1739/1978). *A treatise of human nature*. Oxford: Oxford University Press.

Hursthouse, R. (1999). *On vitue ethics*. Oxford: Oxford University Press.

Jeffrey, D. (2006). *Patient-centred ethics and communication at the end of life*. Oxford: Radcliffe Publishing.

Jeffrey, D. (2014). *Medical mentoring: Supporting students, doctors in training and general practitioners*. London: Royal College of General Practitioners.

Jeffrey, D. (2016). Clarifying empathy: The first step to more humane clinical care. *British Journal of General Practice, 66*, 101–102.

Jeffrey, D. (2017). Communicating with a human voice: Developing a relational model of empathy. *Journal of the Royal College of Physicians of Edinburgh, 47*(3), 267.

Kagan, S. (1998). *Normative ethics*. Boulder, CO: Westview Press.

Kant, I. (1998). *Critique of pure reason*. Cambridge: Cambridge University Press.

Kaplan EA (2011). Empathy and trauma culture: Imagining catastrophe. In A. Coplan & P. Goldie (Eds.), *Empathy: Philosophical and psychological perspectives*. Oxford: Oxford University Press.

Kauppinen, A. (2013). Sentimentalism. In H. LaFollette (Ed.), *International encyclopaedia of ethics*. Oxford: Blackwell.

Kauppinen, A. (2014). Emotion regulation and Moral judgement. In H. Maibom (Ed.), *Empathy and morality*. Oxford: Oxford University Press.

Kearney, M. K., et al. (2009). Self-care of physicians caring for patients at the end of Life "Being Connected.... A Key to Survival". *JAMA, 301*, 1155–1164.

Macnaughton, J. (2009). The dangerous practice of empathy. *Lancet, 373*(9679), 1940–1941.

Maibom, H. L. (2014). (Almost) everything you wanted to know about empathy. In H. L. Maibom (Ed.), *Empathy and morality*. Oxford: Oxford University Press.

Maibom, H. (2017). Empathy and care ethics. In H. L. Maibom (Ed.), *The Routledge handbook of philosophy of empathy* (pp. 264–272). New York: Routledge.

Maibon, H. (2014). *Empathy and morality*. Oxford: Oxford University Press.

Mallia, P. (2013). *The nature of the doctor-patient relationship: Health care principles through the phenomenology of relationships with patients*. Dordrecht: Springer.

Marcum, J. A. (2008). *An introductory philosophy of medicine: Humanizing modern medicine*. Dortrecht: Springer.

Maxwell, B. (2008). *Professional ethics education: Studies in compassionate empathy*. New York: Springer.

Maxwell, B., & Racine, E. (2010). Should empathic development be a priority in biomedical ethics teaching? A critical perspective. *Cambridge Quarterly of Healthcare Ethics, 19*(4), 433–445.

Meyer, M. L., et al. (2013). Empathy for the social suffering of friends and strangers recruits distinct patterns of brain activation. *Scandinavian Audiology, 8*, 446–454.

Meyers, D. T. (1994). *Subjection & subjectivity: Psycoanalytic feminism & moral philosophy*. New York: Routledge.

Miles, S. H. (2005). *The hippocratic oath and the ethics of medicine*. Oxford: Oxford University Press.

Noddings, N. (1984). *Caring: A feminine approach to ethics and moral education*. Berkeley, CA: University of California Press.

Noddings, N. (2013). *Caring: A relational approach to ethics and moral education*. Berkeley, CA: University of California Press.

Oxley, J. C. (2011). *The moral dimensions of empathy limits and applications in ethical theory and practice*. Basingstoke: Palgrave Macmillan.

Pellegrino, E. (1994). The four principles and the doctor-patient relationship: The need for better linkage. In G. R. Chichester (Ed.), *Principles of health care ethics*. John Wiley & Son.

Pellegrino, E. (1999). The origins and evolution of bioethics: Some personal reflections. *Kennedy Institute of Ethics Journal, 9*, 73–88.

Prinz, J. (2011a). Against empathy. *Southern Journal of Philosophy, 49*, 214–233.

Prinz, J. (2011). Is empathy necessary for morality? In A. Coplan & P. Goide (Eds.), *Empathy: Philosophical and psychological approaches*. Oxford: Oxford University Press.

Rawls, J. (2009). *A theory of justice*. Harvard university press.

Rest, J. (1986). An overview of the psychology of morality. In J. Rest (Ed.), *Moral development: Advances in research and theory*. New York: Praeger.

Riess, H. (2015). The impact of clinical empathy on patients and clinicians: Understanding empathy's side effects. *AJOB Neuroscience, 6*(3), 51–53.

Sandel, M. J. (2009). *Justice. What's the right thing to do?* London: Allen Lane.

Scruton, R. (2001). *Kant: A very short introduction.* Oxford: Oxford University Press.

Slote, M. (2007). *The ethics of care and empathy.* London: Routledge.

Smajdor, A., et al. (2011). The limits of empathy: Problems in medical education and practice. *Journal of Medical Ethics, 37*(6), 380–383.

Smith, A. ((1759/1976)). *The theory of moral sentiments.* Oxford: Clarendon.

Sturzu, L., et al. (2019). Empathy and burnout—A cross-sectional study among mental healthcare providers in France. *Journal of Medicine and Life, 12,* 21–29.

Tong, R. (2007). *New perspectives in health care ethics: An interdisciplinary and crosscultural approach.* Upper Saddle River, NJ: Pearson Prentice-Hall.

Tronto, J. C. (1993). *Moral boundaries: A political argument for an ethic of care.* New York: Routledge.

Vagle, M. D. (2016). *Crafting phenomenological research.* London: Routledge.

van Dijke, J., et al. (2019). Care ethics: An ethics of empathy? *Nursing Ethics, 26,* 1282–1291.

Watson, J., & Greenburg, L. (2011). Empathic resonance: A neuroscience perspective. In J. Decety & W. Ickes (Eds.), *The social neuroscience of empathy* (pp. 123–137). London: MIT Press.

Weir, J. M., et al. (2015). From hippocrates to the francis report-reflections on empathy. *The Ulster Medical Journal, 84*(1), 8.

CHAPTER 8

Empathy-Based Ethics in Medical Practice

Abstract The application of the empathy-based ethical approach in clinical practice is examined in three scenarios. Helen's story is described, firstly as a patient with advanced lung cancer receiving hospital-based treatment, then her story is retold with her general practitioner taking a key role in co-ordinating her care. The second case, Peter, is a man with advanced pancreatic cancer who is dying at home. He asks his general practitioner "Will you help me to die, please?" Empathy-based ethics provides a way of responding to a request for euthanasia in a humane and moral way. In the third scenario, the role of the empathy-based approach is examined with reference to the COVID-19 pandemic, looking at the differences between ethical approaches focused on individuals and public health concerns. A relational empathic approach to ethics, acknowledging our interconnection, vulnerability and shared humanity is appropriate to meet the moral challenges of the pandemic.

Keywords Palliative chemotherapy · Euthanasia · Pandemic · Relational autonomy · Empathy-based ethics

INTRODUCTION

This chapter describes the application of an empathy-based ethical framework in clinical practice. The three scenarios used are based on an amalgam of real-life patients' stories with changes in names and gender to preserve confidentiality.

Helen's story is described in two ways, initially as a patient with advanced lung cancer receiving hospital-based treatment from the oncology department. Helen's story is then retold with a different emphasis as her general practitioner takes a key role in co-ordinating her care. The two perspectives illustrate how the approach taken by doctors may dramatically alter the patient experience.

Peter is a man with advanced pancreatic cancer who is dying at home, cared for by his wife and daughter. He asks his general practitioner "Will you help me to die, please?". Empathy-based ethics provides a way of responding to a request for euthanasia in a humane and moral way.

In our account of empathy-based ethics, a strong emphasis has been placed on relational aspects of the patient-doctor relationship. In the third clinical scenario, the role of the empathy-based framework is examined with reference to the COVID-19 pandemic. This case investigates the differences between ethical approaches focused on individuals and public health concerns.

WHAT ARE YOU GOING TO DO NEXT, DOCTOR? CEASING PALLIATIVE CHEMOTHERAPY

Background: Helen's Story

Helen, a 45-year-old non-smoking teacher, is married to Tom, a plumber. They have two children, Charlie and Katie aged 18 and 16. Three weeks ago, Helen developed a dry cough and pains in her lower back. She saw her GP, Dr. Woods, who referred her for X-rays, a scan and blood tests. The results of her investigations showed that Helen had advanced lung cancer with spread to her bones and liver. She was referred to the hospital for further investigation and subsequently referred to Dr. Brown, an oncologist, for chemotherapy (Anandappa and Popat 2016).

HELEN'S STORY: THE BIOMEDICAL APPROACH

Helen met Dr. Brown with her husband in the outpatient clinic. Dr. Brown listened carefully to the history of her symptoms and of her shock of learning that she had lung cancer. She was keen to know what treatment she could have. Dr. Brown explained that her disease would be best treated by a course of chemotherapy which would help her breathlessness and fatigue, and painkillers to relieve her back pain. He explained that chemotherapy would involve coming up to the day-patient ward every three weeks. She would have blood tests and scans to monitor her response to treatment. Helen asked about the side-effects of the chemotherapy and was told of hair-loss and sickness. Helen signed a consent form and Tom confirmed that they both wanted to fight the cancer. Dr. Brown explained that he would write to her GP informing her of the treatment plan. At this initial visit, Helen did not ask about the chance of recovery as Dr Brown appeared busy and the waiting room was full of patients.

Over the course of the next six weeks, Helen felt ill before her chemotherapy, vomited for four days after the drugs and felt tired all the time. She became depressed, withdrawn and her appetite was poor. Her GP, Dr. Woods, left prescriptions for anti-emetics and analgesics for Tom to pick up from the surgery. Reviews at the outpatient clinic focused on the results of blood tests and the treatment plan. Helen became weary of hunting for a car-parking space at the hospital, her whole life seemed to be dominated by her disease and hospital visits.

After two months, a check scan revealed that the disease was progressing. Helen was distraught as she had believed that there was a hope of cure.

Helen complained to Tom, "Dr. Brown would never have put me through all this if there wasn't a good chance of cure".

She was admitted to the ward with increasing pain, breathlessness and low mood. She asked Dr Brown on the ward round,

"What are you going to do next, doctor?"

Dr. Brown explained that her type of lung cancer was not suitable for immunotherapy, but she could try a second-line chemotherapy drug to see if it would help to slow the progress of the disease. Helen said she felt too ill to take any further chemotherapy. Dr. Brown agreed that it would be best if she had a break from treatment and that it would be sensible to see the palliative care team while she was recuperating in the ward.

Helen met the palliative care nurse Morag, but by this time she was very weak, withdrawn and depressed. Morag sat and listened to her and suggested having her drugs for pain and vomiting administered by a syringe pump, which would give her continuous relief from her symptoms. She said she would return in the morning. That night Helen's condition deteriorated rapidly. Tom was called by the night staff, but despite rushing to the hospital with Charlie and Katie, Helen died before they arrived.

Her husband Tom, her children Charlie and Katie were bereft, having no chance to say goodbye in a loving way. Their grief was complicated and prolonged.

DISCUSSION

This version of Helen's story highlights unfortunate outcomes of a strictly biomedical approach to patient care. After being provided with overwhelming amounts of information relating to the cancer, drug treatments and side effects, Helen opts for chemotherapy with the mistaken belief that there is a chance of cure (Aragon 2020).

Conversations during subsequent visits to the clinic were restricted to the details of the treatment plan and results of investigations (The et al. 2000). There was no discussion of Helen's poor prognosis, it remained 'an elephant in the room'. The oncologist did not want to remove hope by raising issues of end of life care, so entered a collusion with the patient (The et al. 2000). He finds conversations about stopping treatment difficult and stressful. Current guidelines set out when to start anticancer treatments, but not when to stop as the end of life approaches (Clarke et al. 2015). Dr. Brown does not routinely involve the palliative care team until the terminal stage of the disease (Aragon 2020).

Helen's general practitioner, Dr. Woods, has handed over her medical care to the oncologist, so has not had any conversations to explore her values and concerns about her cancer. Dr. Woods is doubtful about the value of palliative chemotherapy, but is aware of her own lack of knowledge in this rapidly advancing field (Aragon 2020).

When patients are receiving palliative chemotherapy within the last 30 days of their life questions arise as to the appropriateness of the therapy (Nguyen et al. 2019). There is an increasing trend towards continuing palliative chemotherapy until close to the end of the patient's life (Clarke et al. 2015; Earle et al. 2004; Zdenkowski 2013). The sad consequence in this case is that Helen became depressed, withdrawn and had no chance to discuss her real concerns with her husband Tom, or her children, as her family were drawn into a collusion that she would eventually get better.

Her condition deteriorated suddenly and by this time her professional carers were the hospital staff. She did not have an opportunity to build a relationship with her GP and she did not know the palliative care team. As a result, she was admitted to the hospital and met a palliative care nurse only hours before she died on her own in an oncology ward.

This case demonstrates that the nature of the patient-doctor relationship is a key part of the decision to cease futile chemotherapy (Clarke et al. 2015). Determining when to withhold palliative chemotherapy at the end of life is difficult and emotion becomes an important influence (Bluhm et al. 2016). Some oncologists claim that their decision to continue late chemotherapy is patient-driven. Chemotherapy is sometimes used to palliate emotional distress and maintain patient hope even when physical benefit is unexpected (Bluhm et al. 2016). Oncologists experience stress in emotionally draining communication in a setting of prognostic uncertainty and may respond by offering futile chemotherapy (Bluhm et al. 2016).

HELEN'S STORY: AN EMPATHY-BASED ETHICAL APPROACH

In this scenario, when Dr. Woods met Helen to give her the results of the investigations, she asked Helen about her ideas of the cause of her symptoms. Helen admitted that she was frightened that it might be a cancer, as her mother died of breast cancer. Dr. Woods confirmed that the X-rays showed that she had lung cancer which had also involved her spine and liver. She gave Helen time to express her distress. Helen asked, 'What will happen next?'

Dr. Woods suggested meeting her with her husband the following day when there would be a chance for them to raise questions and to discuss future treatment.

The following afternoon Tom and Helen met Dr. Woods. Helen was keen to know what treatment might offer. Dr. Woods asked her what she expected from treatment and Helen explained that she wanted to feel better, to have less pain and to have as much time as possible at home with Tom and her children.

She asked Dr. Woods, "Am I going to get better?"

Dr. Woods replied, "Before I answer you Helen,please tell me what you think"

Helen looked sad, "I know what happened to my Mum, I know that I am not going to survive this, but how long have I got?"

Dr. Woods replied, "It is very difficult to predict this for any individual, but had you any idea in your mind?"

Helen thought for a moment, "Charlie is going to university in six months and Katie has her GCSE exams this summer so I would like to be here for them"

"Those are realistic goals which we can work together to achieve" said Dr. Woods.

Helen asked, "It would be good to feel less pain and be able to do more, are there things that can help me?"

Dr. Woods explained the importance of taking regular analgesics and suggested involvement of a specialist palliative care nurse. It was also possible that chemotherapy might help some of her symptoms as the goal was to improve her quality of life.

Helen was happy to meet the nurse but looked anxious about the notion of chemotherapy. Dr. Woods reassured her that this would only continue if she was benefiting from it.

Helen said, "It's such a relief to talk about this in the open, Tom and I want the time left together as a family to be special. We will talk to Charlie and Katie this evening and let them know the situation".

Dr. Woods offered to see Charlie and Katie if they had any questions and reassured them that she would keep in touch with Helen and the oncologist Dr. Brown, through her chemotherapy if that was what she chose.

Helen met Dr. Brown with her husband in the outpatient clinic. Dr Brown listened carefully to the history of her symptoms and agreed with her that the focus of treatment of her treatment should be improving her quality of life. He explained that a trial of chemotherapy might help her symptoms of breathlessness, but if it did not then this should stop. Helen was relieved. Dr. Brown asked if she would keep in touch with Dr. Woods and said that he always referred patients in Helen's situation to the palliative care team.

After six weeks, the trial of chemotherapy was not helping her symptoms, so Helen agreed to take a break from the treatment. Dr. Brown introduced Dr. Smith a palliative care specialist who saw Helen and Tom and suggested different analgesics and a small dose of opiate for her breathlessness. Helen also talked about the future and emphasised that she wanted to be at home as much as possible. Dr. Smith said she was available in the background for advice and that her GP and the specialist palliative care nurse would see her regularly at her home.

Helen's pain improved, she managed her breathlessness and felt much less anxious. She was involved in helping Charlie prepare for university and supported Katie through the traumas of GCSE's. Dr. Brown saw her each fortnight and the specialist nurse Maggie each week. Helen found she could talk easily with them and discussed plans for a time when she would be confined to bed. She was gradually getting weaker and after two months found that she was taking a nap in the afternoons.

Her symptoms were well controlled and as she became more tired she asked Dr. Woods on one of her visits,

"When I get more ill will I still be able to stay at home? Can I die at home?"

Dr Brown explained that when the time came there would be extra help and support for her and her family and that they would do everything possible to keep her at home. She asked Helen if she had any particular concerns about the end of her life.

Helen said, "I worry that the breathing, will it get worse will I choke to death?"

Dr Woods reassured Helen by saying that if she became distressed with her breathing she could have sedation which would make her sleepy but not breathless. "You will not choke to death but just become sleepier".

Helen agreed that would be much better and thanked Dr. Woods for her reassurance.

The specialist nurse Maggie helped Helen with her symptom control and with conversations with Charlie and Katie. She also supported Tom as he looked after his dying wife at home.

A month later Helen died peacefully at home with her husband and children around her.

Discussion

In this scenario, Helen and her family were more involved in decisions about her care. From the outset, her GP explored her values and goals of care, which led to agreed aims, improved understanding of prognosis and improved quality of life near the end of life (Aragon 2020).

During the discussion with Helen and Tom, Dr. Woods admitted the difficulty in making a prognosis. He took care to assess how Helen wanted to receive the information. Did she wish statistical information? or as it transpired, did she want to live to see her children through their exams and to reach university? Allowing for silence and being empathic are ways to show support when delivering prognostic information that should be initiated early for patients with advanced lung cancer (Aragon 2020).

Discussions about prognosis may be avoided, as in the first scenario, or be provided in a detrimental way, and like any difficult conversation should be introduced and discussed in a sensitive empathic way (Aragon 2020). Prognosis inherently has a high level of uncertainty, which needs to be acknowledged as Dr. Woods communicated in the second scenario.

Dr. Woods also appropriately suggested early involvement of specialist palliative care. Such early referral in advanced lung cancer has been demonstrated to result in a better quality of life, less depression and less aggressive treatment at the end of life (Temel et al. 2010). These two examples show that if clinicians do not explore the individual's values, a key part of shared decision-making is left out (Aragon 2020). Addressing this early on as in the second scenario sets the tone for future conversations and it makes clear to patients and doctors the importance of values-informed care plans across all stages of lung cancer, and not just for end-of-life decisions (Aragon 2020).

Dr. Woods began what is described as 'advance care planning' from the outset in asking Helen about what was important to her in life and in her medical care. She clarified that she would remain the key health professional managing Helen's care. Dr. Woods took care to discuss and clarify Helen's goals, values, and preferences which were then tailored to her situation, involving her family in the discussions (Aragon 2020). Helen's preferences were reviewed as the disease progressed as her physical condition deteriorated.

As the palliative chemotherapy did not improve her symptoms and did not significantly improve meaningful survival, Dr. Brown was able to feel comfortable in withdrawing treatment. In the second scenario, he prepared Helen for this eventuality and included referral to specialist palliative care in tandem with his treatment, not as a last-minute referral as in the first scenario. Late referral to palliative care occurs because some doctors worry that patients will lose hope or become more depressed if palliative care is discussed. Furthermore, some oncologists may believe that they should be the professionals to provide palliative care (Aragon 2020).

As the disease progressed Helen was at home, in familiar surroundings supported by her family and health professionals she knew and trusted. She was able to discuss difficult issues of her own dying and be reassured by Dr. Woods that she would continue to be supported and receive symptom relief. Patients and their families may have no experience of seeing someone die in their own homes and health professionals are ideally placed to answer their questions and to reassure them that, for most people, dying is a peaceful and dignified process (Mannix 2017).

The second scenario shows how empathy-based ethics places the patient-doctor relationship at its centre, caring for the patient and building trust for future difficult conversations. Uncertainty is a part of clinical medicine but exploration of the patient's values and goals is still possible (Aragon 2020) The initiation of palliative care is much more than a referral process between differing disciplines. It involves the patient and family in readjusting their hopes and expectations and working in partnership with healthcare professionals (Jeffrey and Downie 2003).

In adopting an empathy-based approach, doctors remain mindful of the emotional impact of the situation, adjusting to the different needs of different patients (and their families). They clearly demonstrate a collaborative approach with the patient and try to understand how the patient perceives the situation, rather than how they do (Owen and Jeffrey 2008). The empathic nature of the patient-doctor relationship is a key part of decision-making concerning the withdrawal of anticancer drugs towards the end of life, supporting the importance on 'trust' and 'empathy' in shared healthcare decision-making (Kraetschmer et al. 2004). Time spent with patients and their families is worthwhile work for doctors (Jeffrey 2000).

PLEASE WILL YOU HELP ME TO DIE?: A REQUEST FOR EUTHANASIA

Background; Peter's Story

Peter, a 65-year-old retired builder is married to Joan, they have an unmarried daughter Lucy, aged 40. Peter had been treated for depression over the past three months by his general practitioner Dr. Strang. Four weeks ago, Peter developed sudden severe abdominal pain and was admitted to hospital where a pancreatic cancer with liver metastases was diagnosed. The cancer was inoperable and Peter did not wish any palliative chemotherapy, so was discharged home after two weeks. Lucy has taken leave from her job as a librarian to help her mother at home to look after Peter. Peter and the family were informed by the surgeon in hospital that the prognosis was poor and that he might have "a few months to live".

Peter has severe abdominal pain and is receiving opiate analgesics through a syringe pump. He is visited each day by a district nurse and spends most of the time confined to his room sitting in a chair or resting in bed. His general practitioner Dr. Strang visits him to review his pain control. Peter tells him that he feels low, his pain keeps him awake and he cannot see much point in going on. He looks to Dr. Strang and asks him, "Will you help me to die, please?".

Dr. Strang paused "That is a very difficult question, can we talk about things?"

He sat beside Peter in silence.

Peter began to weep, "I know that I'm going to die and it's going to be agony. I don't want to be a burden to Joan and Lucy. Wouldn't it just be better to give me an injection to end my suffering now?"

Dr. Strang replied, "This must be very difficult for you, what is it that troubles you most?"

Peter answered, "It's being a burden, I have always been independent, the strong one, now Joan and Lucy are having to look after me. My wife has become my nurse".

Dr. Strang said, "That must be hard for you to accept. What would you have done if it was Joan who was ill and you were well?"

"I would have looked after her of course, I would have wanted to" replied Peter.

"Well, maybe that is how it is for Joan and Lucy. They love you, want to be close to you and care for you at this difficult time" said Dr. Strang.

Peter sat quietly "I had not thought of it like that".

Dr. Strang said "You mentioned dying in agony Peter, is that another worry?"

Peter replied, "Yes, I saw my grandfather die many years ago, he was groaning in pain, no one gave him any pain relief"

Dr. Strang explained, "There have been huge advances in pain control since then. I can promise you that we will work together to get on top of your pain. You must tell me or the district nurse if you have any pain and we can adjust the dose of drugs to suit you. I am so glad you have talked about your concerns Peter. I just wonder if there are any things you would like to do in the time that is left?"

"Well doctor, I would love to see some of my friends, they have stayed away because they don't know what to say to me. Joan and I love the countryside, it would be lovely to have a visit to the river side. Lucy has just moved to a new flat and as a builder I would love to get a look at it".

"These are all sensible aims Peter, let us get Joan and Lucy into discuss how we can achieve this. The district nurse can arrange a wheelchair and the ambulance men are happy to lift you up to the flat one afternoon. But before I leave, are you still wanting to end your life?" asked Dr. Strang.

"No, I was just so low and you have made me think that there is a point in going on. I feel much happier that you and the nurses will make sure that I won't suffer when the end comes. I want to say Dr. Strang that we are all grateful for your care. They told me at the hospital how pancreatic cancer can sometimes appear as depression and physical symptoms only appear at a late stage"

"Thank you, Peter, I must admit I felt guilty that I might have missed something when the letter from the hospital came. We have had a good talk today and we can make a start planning for some of the things you have raised. I will be back next week but you have my number, I am happy to visit if you need me before that".

After this conversation, Peter's mood brightened, the dose of analgesics could be reduced and his pain settled. He and Joan and Lucy were closer and enjoyed visits to the park. Lucy was grateful to her father for his advice on some alterations necessary in her flat. Friends visited and reminisced about the happy times they had shared. Peter realised that he was valued in spite of his poor physical state. After six weeks, he died peacefully at home.

DISCUSSION

Sensitive exploration of a request for euthanasia or physician-assisted suicide can reveal the real needs of the patient (Jeffrey 2006). The request for euthanasia points to a number of concerns that the patient has about dying; loss of self, loss of dignity and the social context of dying. It may take time to understand all the reasons behind the request, continuity of care is important in developing such an empathic relationship.

In Peter's case, the patient-doctor relationship deepened as Dr. Strang sat quietly and listened to his concerns. He knew that he was not legally allowed to carry out euthanasia, but stating this at the outset might have alienated Peter (Jeffrey 2009). Dr. Strang acknowledged Peter's distress, elicited concerns and then discovered goals that Peter wanted to achieve which would improve his quality of life and reassure him that he was still valued.

He also returned in the conversation to check if Peter still had a wish to shorten his life. As their relationship deepened, Peter thanked his GP and forgave him for the delay in diagnosis, evidence of a deep empathy as Dr Strang then was able to share his own vulnerability.

Once psychological issues are addressed, the requirement for analgesics often reduces since anxiety and depression exacerbate pain. Peter was much brighter once he appreciated that he was valued by his friends and could still contribute to his family. He mattered to the very end of his life (Chochinov 2007).

EMPATHY-BASED ETHICS IN RESPONSE TO THE COVID-19 PANDEMIC

Introduction

The coronavirus or COVID-19 pandemic presents ethical challenges for patients, their families, healthcare workers, policymakers and the public. Responding to a public health crisis of this nature demands a broader relational ethical perspective than the four-principle approach of traditional medical ethics (Beauchamp and Childress 2013; Jeffrey 2020). Clinical and research ethics has traditionally focused on the individual whereas public health ethics addresses the interests of a population (Thompson et al. 2006). This shift in ethical focus is one which most healthcare workers struggle with since clinicians are trained to adopt a duty-based ethical approach, placing the individual patient at the centre of care. When health risks primarily affect an individual, respect for autonomy has a high value. However, when a population is at risk, collective interests assume a greater relevance (Baylis et al. 2008). Harsh utilitarian values may be softened by adopting relational ethical values; solidarity, duty, equity, relational autonomy, trust and reciprocity. It is essential that particular attention is paid to the socially or economically disadvantaged, in order to achieve the best possible outcomes since these groups are most at risk (World Health Organisation 2007).

Isolation and Social Distancing

Isolation and social distancing impose limits on an individual's freedom and autonomy to maximise the welfare of society (World Health Organisation 2007). The principle of reciprocity is relevant since in a situation where an individual's rights are limited, the government has a reciprocal duty to limit any consequent burdens on the individual (Shearer 2020). In particular, the needs of vulnerable groups including; racial and ethnic minorities, elderly people, prisoners, disabled persons, migrants and the homeless should be of the greatest priority (Baylis et al. 2008; World Health Organisation 2007). The burdens of social isolation include loneliness, uncertainty, stress, depression and anxiety and even death (Roy et al. 2020). Other mental health problems arising from prolonged isolation include addiction, domestic violence and post-traumatic stress disorder (Roy et al. 2020). Grieving in isolation may be prolonged for families unable to visit their dying relative (Moore 2020).

Personal protective equipment including face masks distance healthcare professionals and families from patients. Contact between patients and their families may be limited to video calls or the telephone. Developing close empathic relationships with such barriers may be challenging, doctors need time to be present with patients and to be able to communicate their concern despite having to wear face masks (Schlogl 2020).

If the measures to limit the spread of the disease are to be successful, the authorities need the public's trust (Brody and Avery 2009). A continuing dialogue is needed between health professionals, government and society to maintain trust and solidarity.

Relational Autonomy

We are all dependent upon others, the interests of the individual and community are inevitably inter-related. Autonomy should adopt a relational form which takes account of the effects of exercising one's autonomy on the autonomy of others (Dworkin 1988; Mackenzie and Stoljar 2001). Relational autonomy involves a change in emphasis from the individual self to a person embedded in a social context (Mackenzie and Stoljar 2001). This contrasts with the current view of autonomy which stresses independence and self-interest (Dworkin 1988).

Solidarity

To achieve social distancing and voluntary self-isolation of large numbers of affected or vulnerable people requires the ethical concept of solidarity; where individuals are firmly united by common responsibilities and interests (World Health Organisation 2007). Solidarity involves relational empathy and virtues such as altruism, kindness and generosity, extending to include the concept of fellowship (Brody and Avery 2009; Jeffrey 2016a, b). Solidarity is a relational construct, reflecting a shared interest in survival and safety, a feeling of "we are all in this together" (Baylis et al. 2008).

Healthcare Workers' Duty of Care to Patients

Doctors and nurses have a fundamental duty of care, so cannot, with integrity, refuse to care for patients with COVID-19 (Brody and Avery 2009). However, healthcare workers are assumed to adopt a view that their duty to care overrides self-preservation, consequently there is little debate about any limits to this duty of care (Brody and Avery 2009). A doctor's moral obligation to work is not unlimited; factors such as the risks to the doctor and their family, competing family caregiving responsibilities and duties of care to other patients must be taken into account (World Health Organisation 2007). The duty of care is linked to the ethics of solidarity between NHS workers and members of society. Some doctors have died in the course of treating patients with COVID-19, so it appears that the duty to care is not dependent upon the extent of risk (Brody and Avery 2009).

Social Obligations: Solidarity and Reciprocity

Solidarity between health professionals and society is a key ethical value in minimising mortality and morbidity in a pandemic (Brody and Avery 2009). Society grants professionals privileges and respect and in a reciprocal way expects them to care for infectious patients. Politically, solidarity is endorsed by the authorities appealing to a concept of relational empathy and supporting healthcare workers (Jeffrey 2016b).

Reciprocal moral obligations exist on the part of governments and employers to protect and support healthcare professionals working during the pandemic (World Health Organisation 2007). Healthcare workers should not be expected to expose themselves to unnecessary risk where employers have not provided appropriate personal protective equipment (PPE) (British Medical Association 2020).

Access to Treatment When Resources are Limited: Utility and Equity

When considering rationing of resources from a utilitarian perspective, the ethical goal is to save as many lives as possible. However, this utility principle must be aligned with equity, the distribution of resources should be fair. Fairness through impartiality means that where life and health are involved, every individual, irrespective of age, wealth, gender, status, religion, political opinions, or merits has the same dignity, the same moral value and, therefore, the right to equal treatment in case of illness (Federal Office of Public Health 2018). Nobody should receive privileged medical treatment at the expense of other affected individuals on the basis of their ability to pay, their standing, their social position or their age (Federal Office of Public Health 2018).

DISCUSSION

The poor and socially disadvantaged bear the brunt of the tough public health measures which have been introduced to contain the spread of the virus (Baker 2020). The COVID-19 pandemic is a global disaster which has exposed social realities in our communities (Baker 2020). Brody claims that our response to pandemics prompts us to question, "What sort of society do we want to live in?" (Brody and Avery 2009). A relational empathic approach to ethics, acknowledging our interconnection, vulnerability and shared humanity is appropriate to meet the moral challenges of the pandemic (Jeffrey 2020). Autonomy becomes an ethical construct with responsibilities to other members of society rather than a manifestation of selfishness.

Conclusions

This chapter illustrates the empathy-based approach to ethics in clinical practice. The two individual case histories show how an empathy based-approach reveals deeper levels of information once the patient is allowed to express their values and concerns. In an empathic relationship, the patient becomes involved in their management and gains a sense of control in situations of great uncertainty. The final scenario describes how a relational empathy-based approach may be appropriate in meeting the ethical challenges of a pandemic. The next chapter examines how the empathy-based ethical approach can be embedded in practice, education and research.

References

Anandappa, G., & Popat, S. (2016). Management of lung cancer. *Medicine, 44,* 244–246.

Aragon, K. N. (2020). Palliative care in lung cancer. *Clinics in Chest Medicine, 41,* 281–293.

Baker, P. (2020, 31 March 2020). We can't go back to normal; how will the coronavirus change the world? *The Guardian.* From https://www.thegua rdian.com/world/2020/mar/31/how-will-the-world-emerge-from-the-cor onavirus-crisis.

Baylis, F., Kenny, N. P., & Sherwin, S. (2008). A relational account of public health ethics. *Public Health Ethics, 1*(3), 196–209.

Beauchamp, T., & Childress, J. (2013). *Principles of biomedical ethics.* New York: Oxford University Press.

Bluhm, M., Connell, C. M., De Vries, R. G., Janz, N. K., Bickel, K. E., & Silveira, M. J. (2016). Paradox of prescribing late chemotherapy: oncologists explain. *Journal of Oncology Practice, 12*(12), e1006–e1015.

British Medical Association. (2020). *COVID-19 Ethical issues. A guidance note.* Retrieved 3 April 2020, from https://www.bma.org.uk/media/2226/bma-covid-19-ethics-guidance.pdf.

Brody, H., & Avery, E. N. (2009). Medicine's duty to treat pandemic illness: Solidarity and vulnerability. *Hastings Center Report, 39*(1), 40–48.

Chochinov, H. (2007). Dignity and the essence of medicine: The A, B, C, and D of dignity conserving care. *BMJ, 335,* 184–187.

Clarke, G., Johnston, S., Corrie, P., Kuhn, I., & Barclay, S. (2015). Withdrawal of anticancer therapy in advanced disease: A systematic literature review. *BMC Cancer, 15,* 892–891.

Dworkin, G. (1988). *The concept of autonomy*. Cambridge: Cambridge University Press.

Earle, C. C., Neville, B. A., Landrum, M. B., Ayanian, J. Z., Block, S. D., & Weeks, J. C. (2004). Trends in the aggressiveness of cancer care near the end of life. *Journal of Clinical Oncology, 22*(2), 315–321.

Federal Office of Public Health. (2018). *The Swiss Influenza Pandemic Plan.* from https://www.bag.admin.ch/bag/en/home/das-bag/publikationen/broschueren/publikationen-uebertragbare-krankheiten/pandemieplan-2018.html.

Jeffrey, D. (2000). *Cancer: From cure to care*. Hochland and Hochland: Manchester.

Jeffrey, D. (2006). *Patient-centred ethics and communication at the end of life.* Oxford: Radcliffe Publishing.

Jeffrey, D. (2009). *Against physician assisted suicide*. Oxford: Radcliffe Publishing Ltd.

Jeffrey, D. (2016a). A duty of kindness. *Journal of the Royal Society of Medicine, 109*(7), 261–263.

Jeffrey, D. (2016b). Empathy, sympathy and compassion in healthcare: Is there a problem? Is there a difference? does it matter? *Journal Royal Society Medicine, 109*, 446–452.

Jeffrey, D. (2020). Relational ethical approaches to the COVID-19 pandemic. *Journal Medical Ethics, 46*, 495–498.

Jeffrey, D., & Owen, R. (2003). Changing the emphasis from active curative care to active palliative care in haematology patients. In S. Booth, E. Bruera & J. Craig (Eds.), *Palliative care consultations in haemato-oncology*. Oxford: Oxford University Press.

Kraetschmer, N., Sharpe, N., Urowitz, S., & Deber, R. B. (2004). How does trust affect patient preferences for participation in decision-making? *Health Expectations, 7*(4), 317–326.

Mackenzie, C., & Stoljar, N. (2001). *Relational autonomy*. Oxford: Oxford University Press.

Mannix, K. (2017). *With the end in mind: Death dying and wisdom in an age of denial*. London: William Collins.

Moore, B. (2020). Dying during Covid-19. *Hastings Center Report, 50*, 13–15.

Nguyen, M., et al. (2019). Anticancer therapy within the last 30 days of life: Results of an audit and re-audit cycle from an Australian regional cancer centre. *Journal of Clinical Oncology, 37*, e18260–e18260.

Owen, R., & Jeffrey, D. (2008). Communication: Common challenging scenarios in cancer care. *European Journal of Cancer, 44*, 1163–1168.

Roy, J., Jain, R., Golamari, R., Vunnam, R., & Sahu, N. (2020). COVID-19 in the geriatric population. *International Journal of Geriatric Psychiatry, 1*, 1–5.

Schlogl, M. (2020). Maintaining our humanity through the mask: Mindful communication during Covid-19. *Journal of American Geriatric Society, 68,* E12–E13.

Shearer, J. (2020). *Coronavirus and the ethics of quarantine-why information matters.* from https://blogs-bmj-com.ezproxy.is.ed.ac.uk/bmj/2020/02/17/coronavirus-and-the-ethics-of-quarantine-why-information-matters/.

Temel, J. S., Greer, J. A., Muzikansky, A., Gallagher, E. R., Admane, S., Jackson, V. A., ... & Billings, J. A. (2010). Early palliative care for patients with metastatic non–small-cell lung cancer. *New England Journal of Medicine, 363*(8), 733–742.

The, A.-M., Hak, T., Koëter, G., & van der Wal, G. (2000). Collusion in doctor-patient communication about imminent death: An ethnographic study. *Bmj, 321*(7273), 1376–1381.

Thompson, A. K., Faith, K., Gibson, J. L., & Upshur, R. E. (2006). Pandemic influenza preparedness: An ethical framework to guide decision-making. *BMC Medical Ethics, 7*(1), 12.

World Health Organisation. (2007). *Ethical considerations in developing a public health response to pandemic influenza.* Geneva: World Health Organization.

Zdenkowski, N., Cavenagh, J., Ku, Y. C., Bisquera, A., & Bonaventura, A. (2013). Administration of chemotherapy with palliative intent in the last 30 days of life: The balance between palliation and chemotherapy. *Internal Medicine Journal, 43*(11), 1191–1198.

CHAPTER 9

Embedding Empathy-Based Ethics into Practice, Education and Research

Abstract Empathy-based ethics centres on the patient-doctor relationship, embracing both cognitive and affective aspects. The polarities between biomedical and psychosocial aspects of practice disappear as both are considered to be of importance. Evidence-based medicine becomes integrated with empathy-based ethics. The biomedical gaze switches to a phenomenological approach to care. The medical education literature indicates that empathy can be enhanced or facilitated. An empathy-based approach suggests that a more useful line of research would be to explore the patient-doctor relationship empathy by qualitative methods. The following measures may help to embed empathy in clinical care: clarifying definitions, redressing the imbalance between biomedical and psychological approaches to care, incorporating phenomenology and supporting doctors. Educational initiatives to foster medical students' empathy include: awareness of the importance of empathy, increasing patient contact, guidance on boundary setting, encouraging reflection, mentoring, an empathic learning culture, positive role models, providing support and incorporating the humanities into the curriculum.

Keywords Empathy-based ethics · Evidence-based medicine · Phenomenology · Medical humanities · Medical education

© The Author(s), under exclusive license to Springer Nature
Switzerland AG 2020
D. I. Jeffrey, *Empathy-Based Ethics*,
https://doi.org/10.1007/978-3-030-64804-6_9

INTRODUCTION

This chapter examines how empathy-based ethics may be embedded into clinical practice, medical education and research. Empathy-based ethics centres on the patient-doctor relationship and takes account of the context of the encounter. Empathy conceptualised in broad terms, embraces both cognitive and affective aspects. The polarities between biomedical and psychosocial dissolve as both aspects of medicine are considered to be of importance. Evidence-based medicine becomes integrated with empathy-based ethics. The biomedical gaze switches to a phenomenological approach to care. Phenomenology describes both a philosophy and a research approach (Finlay 2013). Phenomenology aims at gaining a deeper understanding of the meaning of the patient's experiences as they are lived (Van Manen 2016). It has been described as a way of seeing how things appear to us through experience, from another individual's perspective(Carel 2016). Phenomenology claims that any effort to understand the patient's world has to be grounded in their experience of social reality.

Embedding empathy into practice also requires attention to the clinical context. It is not sufficient to train medical students and doctors to practice empathically and expect them to work sensitively in situations where they are stressed, lack time or receive little support.

There is some debate in the medical education literature as to whether empathy can be taught (Jeffrey and Downie 2016). At the heart of the medical undergraduate learning experience is the patient-student relationship. If this is to be an effective relationship, students need to be encouraged to build an empathic dialogue with patients (Jeffrey 2018). The medical education literature indicates that empathy can be enhanced or facilitated in a number of ways, but a lack of long term studies makes it difficult to know whether these effects are sustained (Jeffrey 2018). Empathy's role in ethical functioning is underestimated in standard "judgement-focused" approaches to biomedical ethics education (Maxwell and Racine 2010). A number of innovative approaches to enhancing empathy-based ethics in medical education are discussed (Maxwell 2008).

Medical research into empathy is dominated by quantitative studies trying to measure empathy (Pedersen 2009). In focusing on empathy as an attribute of the doctor rather than an experience within a relationship such research risks losing sight of the main aim of medical education research which is to improve patient care (Cleland 2015). An empathy-based approach suggests that a more useful line of research in the future would be to explore empathy by qualitative methods looking at the patient-doctor relationship. Phenomenology, with its emphasis on empathy, is the ideal research methodology to adopt in such studies (Smith et al. 2009).

EMBEDDING EMPATHY-BASED ETHICS IN CLINICAL PRACTICE

The following measures may help to embed empathy in clinical care:

Clarifying Empathy

The first step in embedding empathy-based ethics into clinical practice is to clarify and agree a concept of empathy. I have argued for a broad relational view of empathy as the foundation of medical ethics which takes account of the context (Jeffrey 2016a, 2017). There has unfortunately been a tendency in undergraduate medical education to present empathy in isolation, as something different from clinical understanding (Foster and Freeman 2008; Pedersen 2010; Shapiro 2008). However, relational empathy is integral to effective clinical medicine. Pedersen explained that such empathy was needed to understand a patient's illness, their emotional reactions to it and to ascertain what is most important to them, in order to diagnose and treat them appropriately (Pedersen 2010).

Balancing the Biomedical and Psychosocial Dimensions of Care

There is a need to redress the imbalance between biomedical and psychological approaches to care. Employing an empathy-based ethical approach to clinical decision-making ensures that the patient's experience of their illness, their concerns and values must be taken into account. It has been suggested that clinical medicine be seen as an interpretative practice rather than as a pure science (Montgomery 2006).

Incorporating Phenomenology

One of the aims of empathy-based ethics is to create a culture of medical practice which acknowledges both biomedical and psychosocial dimensions, leading to a more humane form of care. Clinical practice and phenomenology share characteristics; a willingness to try and see the world from the other person's point of view and a commitment to reflexivity. Thirty years ago Schon argued that there was a need to incorporate phenomenology into teaching and clinical practice, other researchers have echoed his call (Carel 2016; Montgomery 2006; Schön 1987; Vagle 2010; Van Manen 2016).

By incorporating phenomenology into the medical culture, students and doctors would be enabled to use their innate empathic concern and clinical curiosity to empathise with patients, exploring with them the meaning of their illness. A philosophical foundation of phenomenology embraces openness and uncertainty, so fostering such empathy. Such an approach accepts imperfection and by adopting a patient-centred relational approach, allows doctors to connect more closely with patients (Shapiro 2008). A shared willingness to feel and convey empathy may result in a culture shift in medicine from detached concern to adopting a broad view of empathy as a dynamic relational process.

Provide Support for Doctors

A recent GMC report identified that doctors in the UK report considerable work pressure, poor psychological well-being and stress (General Medical Council 2019). A systematic review of psychiatric morbidity in doctors revealed a prevalence rate of psychiatric disorders to range from 17 to 52% (Imo UO 2017). A report from Birbeck concluded that "it is crucial to provide doctors with more support from recruitment to retirement and develop a culture that challenges the mental health stigma and encourages help seeking" (Kinman and Teoh 2018) .

A heavy clinical workload and shortage of time may lead to reduced empathy, clinical errors and further stress (Ahrweiler et al. 2014). There are a number of quantitative studies which show that burnout is associated with a decline in empathy (Brazeau et al. 2010; Paro et al. 2014; Shanafelt et al. 2005). The literature suggests that empathy prevents burnout since it is claimed that emotionally engaged physicians were fulfilled and so had greater effectiveness (Halpern 2001). Doctors need support throughout their careers and time should be made available for mentoring, for all doctors, not just those found to be struggling (Jeffrey 2014).

EMPATHY-BASED ETHICS IN MEDICAL EDUCATION

Can Empathy-Based Ethics Be Taught?

There is a debate in the literature whether empathy can be taught (Davis, 1990; Shapiro 2012; Underman and Hirshfield 2016) . Downie argues that empathy should not be taught, since feelings might impair sound clinical judgement, maintaining that a doctor's friendly manner was sufficient, while others suggest that enhancing empathy was a high priority (Georgi et al. 2014; Jeffrey and Downie 2016; Kiosses et al. 2016; Pedersen 2010).

A number of literature reviews conclude that educational interventions could increase medical student empathy (Batt-Rawden et al. 2013; Kelm et al. 2014; Pedersen 2010; Stepien and Baernstein 2006). Authors have recommended that medical educators should consider using relationship-centred care as a foundation for their interventions to teach empathy (Batt-Rawden et al. 2013).

Interventions to Enhance Empathy in Medical Education

Reinforce the Importance of Empathy

From recruitment, medical students need to be aware of the fundamental importance of empathy in clinical care. Their awareness might be increased by including empathy as an outcome of the formal curriculum. Medical educators could help to emphasise empathy by identifying empathic consultations and giving students positive feedback. At present, some students report a lack of emphasis on empathy in their teaching, which they interpret as a reflection of its unimportance to the medical faculty (Jeffrey 2018; Woloschuk et al. 2004).

Encourage Face-to-Face Contact with Patients

A relational view of empathy prioritises the patient's experience as a source of learning. Students say that patient contact is the most influential factor in enhancing their empathy (Egnew and Wilson 2010; Jeffrey 2018; Tavakol et al. 2012; Winseman et al. 2009). A decline in bedside teaching and a greater emphasis on simulation both for teaching and assessment of clinical skills may contribute to inhibiting students empathising with patients (Elder and Verghese 2015).

Psychosocial issues and empathy could be addressed in the context of a relationship between the student and the patient, with mentoring from an experienced doctor rather than in didactic teaching (Monrouxe et al. 2011). Other initiatives could include a greater emphasis on the patient experience during the lectures and patient involvement with problem-based learning which then becomes patient-based learning (Bleakley and Bligh 2008). A lack of continuity of contact with patients risks the development of detachment (Montgomery 2006). Students also have identified a lack of exposure to patients from ethnic minority groups, different cultures and LGBT people (Jeffrey 2018).

Acknowledge the Limitations of Using Simulated Patients to Foster Empathy
Students stressed that contact with real patients rather than actors, or simulated patients, enhanced their empathy (Egnew and Wilson 2010; Jeffrey 2018). There may be a risk that the use of simulated patients to teach communication skills may lead to the development of 'fake' empathy (Hooker 2015). Communication skills training often involves simulated patient encounters, in which a trained lay person role-plays a patient (Underman 2015). Authors have pointed to the limitation of teaching empathy with simulated patients (Bleakley and Bligh 2008; Wear and Varley 2008). They have argued that there is a risk that if communication with the patient is taught simply as a skill to be acquired and assessed, then resulting relationships with patients may be shallow and mechanistic (Marshall and Bleakley 2009). However, others have pointed out that if the students can imagine that the experience is real, such teaching gave them an opportunity to practice empathy in a safe environment (Underman 2015). A tension exists between authenticity and artificiality, both the simulated patient and the student may just put on a performance rather than empathising (Perrella 2016). If empathy cannot exist in this artificial environment, it casts doubt on the validity of assessing empathy in an OSCE situation with simulated patients (Perrella 2016). Authors reflect that true empathy is not a simulation, nor simply a competence, but a treasure to have and to receive, revealing a transcendent quality to empathy (Wear and Varley 2008).

Restore a Balance Between Biomedical and Psychosocial Elements of Care

Students learn that empathy is not valued as much as biomedical learning and the technical aspects of treatment and evidence-based medicine (EBM) (Jeffrey 2018). Medicine's identification with science appears to offer students and doctors a way of avoiding emotions and their implicit danger of subjectivity (Montgomery 2006). The biomedical emphasis, in excluding psychosocial elements of care, promotes objectivity and detachment from patients (Halpern 2001; Pedersen 2010). Hardy warned that the suppression of empathy may become seen as a desirable skill for a physician (Hardy 2017). Such physicians, who embody the scientific attitude, can be role models for students who then risk losing empathy with patients (Hardy 2017). It seems therefore, that adopting the scientific biomedical model exclusively can contribute to detachment and a lack of empathy. Forty years ago, in a seminal paper advocating a biopsychosocial approach to medicine, Engel wrote, "Nothing will change unless or until those who control resources have the wisdom to venture off the beaten path of exclusive reliance on biomedicine as the only approach to health care" (Engel 1977).

A strong biomedical emphasis in the curriculum seems to have two main effects on students: it causes them distress by neglecting psychosocial aspects of the patient's suffering and it distances them from patients (Jeffrey 2018; Sheikh et al. 2013). There is a need to give psychosocial care the same value as the scientific elements of the curriculum to balance evidence-based medicine with empathy-based medicine. Medical education, and clinical practice, needs to integrate both the science and humanity of patient care by encouraging students to express empathy with patients (Cohen and Sherif 2014).

Balancing Detachment and Connection: Giving Guidance on Setting Appropriate Boundaries

Research suggests that students struggle to empathise because they do not know how to regulate their emotions (Eikeland et al. 2014; Jeffrey 2018; Ratanawongsa et al. 2005). Most students want to be both competent and empathic but are uncertain how to balance an emotional connection with the patient with detachment in their clinical decision-making (Eikeland et al. 2014). Detached concern prevails in the medical culture despite the fact that there is little evidence that establishing an emotional connection with a patient leads to a negative outcome (Halpern 2001; Jeffrey 2018;

120   D. I. JEFFREY

Montgomery 2006). Emotional insights can and should inform clinical decision-making (Coulehan 1995; Halpern 2001; Kozlowski et al. 2017; Mayer et al. 2008).

There is little discussion in the wider medical education literature about how students might manage their emotions (Coulehan 1995; Meier et al. 2001). If students are to connect emotionally with patients they need the support and guidance of experienced doctors (Ballatt and Campling 2011; Bleakley and Bligh 2008).

There is a lack of understanding of the distinction between appropriate empathetic concern and harmful personal distress (Decety and Meyer 2008). In relational empathy, the student or doctor is emotionally engaged with the patient and at same time is able to reflect on the emotions, knowing that they originate in the other person (Halpern 2001). However, if a self-orientated perspective is taken by the student, the result is personal distress and distancing from the patient (Ekman and Halpern 2015).

Encouraging Reflection with a Mentor
Students value an opportunity to be able to talk to a patient, reflect and receive feedback without feeling that they were being assessed (Janssen et al. 2008; Jeffrey 2018). Students also describe reflection as a strategy for coping with stress, and so enhancing their empathy (Jeffrey 2018). Awareness of the self, of the other and of the relational space between the two are key objectives for reflective approaches to cultivate empathy.

Providing students with a space for dialogue may be one way of nurturing reflection, empathy and of reducing stress (Branch 2010; Lutz et al. 2013; Ramesh 2013). Empathy has a spatial dimension, the closer the contact both physically and emotionally to the patient the deeper the empathy. It seems that this close contact is balanced by a need to pause, to step back to allow reflection on the patient's experience, moving between the specific individual and drawing on wider past experience.

Fostering an Empathic Learning Culture
The students' experience of their learning environment may be described as the culture of the medical school (Genn 2001). Students perceive that they occupy a low position in the hierarchy of the medical school and experience a pressure to compete (Lempp and Seale 2004; Ratanawongsa et al. 2005). They described situations where showing feelings was

discouraged by senior doctors, with the result that students became reluctant to show emotions (Eikeland et al. 2014). Instead, students linked their need to be professional with detachment from patients (Tavakol et al. 2012). Empathy should be seen as essential to clinical practice not as something 'nice' but irrelevant to 'real' medicine (Jeffrey and Downie 2016).

Hafferty (1998), described three parts of the learning environment: the formal curriculum (which is stated and formally intended), the informal curriculum (which is ad hoc interpersonal teaching between faculty and students) and the hidden curriculum (which is a set of influences that occur in organisational culture involving understandings, customs and rituals) (Lempp and Seale 2004). In a study of the hidden curriculum, authors identified positive role models, haphazard teaching, hierarchy and competition as themes determining the medical school culture(Lempp and Seale 2004).

Some students claim that they are not shown empathy by the medical school, citing harsh attitudes of teaching staff to sickness absence and bereavement indicating that the medical school treated them, at times, with suspicion rather than as colleagues needing support (Jeffrey 2018). Other authors have made the case for students needing more empathy from the faculty and their teachers before they can truly understand how to establish empathetic connections (Bayne 2011; Janssen and MacLeod 2010; Karnieli-Miller et al. 2011). A recent study showed how curricular change, in this case introduction of small group work and academic communities, enhanced the students' sense of connection with faculty (Brandl et al. 2017).

A competitive culture in the medical school is not conducive to developing empathy and may risk patient care (Lempp and Seale 2004; Marcum 2013; Nogueira-Martins et al. 2006).The hierarchy within a medical school contributes to a conforming culture (Lempp and Seale 2004). Students are distressed to observe doctors behaving without empathy but feel constrained from challenging a consultant's behaviour (Monrouxe and Rees 2012; Rees and Monrouxe 2011; Rees et al. 2013). Abuse of power by humiliation or bullying undermines students' confidence and empathy with patients (Lempp and Seale 2004). Commonly students take no action in response to bullying (Rees and Monrouxe 2011). It appears that awareness by the medical faculty of abuse of students in medical education has resulted in little effective change (Rees and Monrouxe 2011; Timm 2014).

Medical teachers also need to have time allocated for teaching, which should be recognised and valued by the administration(Pedersen 2010). The successful integration of empathy-based ethics into medical undergraduate education demands that the student lives within an environment that values and engages empathically. It is not sufficient simply to insert a course on empathy but rather the empathy-based ethical approach needs to be integrated throughout the curriculum. It will be successful when the hidden curriculum mirrors the importance of empathy-based ethics. The challenge is to transform institutional culture creating an empathic, ethical institution.

Provide Positive Role Models
Positive, caring role models are an effective way of learning to empathise with patients (Cutler et al. 2009; Lempp and Seale 2004; Nogueira-Martins et al. 2006). Conversely, students are distressed by negative role models, doctors who appear insensitive, and lacking an interest in patients' psychosocial concerns (Lempp and Seale 2004; Nogueira-Martins et al. 2006; Ratanawongsa et al. 2005). Students also highlight the stressful effect of humiliation and bullying by poor role models (Lempp and Seale 2004).

A lack of positive role models has been suggested as a factor in causing students to have unrealistic expectations of how a doctor should behave (Chen et al. 2007). It has also been suggested that academic staff no longer build their reputations on clinical teaching expertise but are now judged on their ability to secure research grants and publish scientific papers (Elder and Verghese 2015).

Students appreciated when experienced doctors admitted their vulnerability and showed emotions (Jeffrey 2018). This was in contrast to the generally accepted notion that the expression of emotions by doctors was a sign of weakness or incompetence (Kerasidou and Horn 2016). Students claimed that when their teachers explicitly shared the emotional aspects of a situation it was a powerful way of learning (Passi et al. 2013). Another study in the USA found excellent role models were those who stressed the importance of the doctor-patient relationship and taught psychosocial aspects of medicine (Wright et al. 1998).

Providing Support and Reducing Stress
Student distress contributes to cynicism and subsequently affects patient care and the culture of the medical profession (Dyrbye et al. 2005).There

is abundant evidence that workplace stress in healthcare organisations affects quality of care for patients as well as doctors' own health (West and Coia 2019). Social support and a plan for self-care are essential for maintaining physical and mental health with lack of support being a risk factor for psychological illness (Sanchez-Reilly et al. 2013) (Cacioppo et al. 2011; George and Gerada 2019; Ozbay et al. 2007; Reblin and Uchino 2008). Medical students and doctors need to develop effective mechanisms of self-care and healthy ways of relieving stress to maintain their well-being (Coulehan and Williams; Kerasidou and Horn 2016).

Since students identify stress as a prominent inhibitor of empathy the provision of support for students would appear to be essential. Providing support for medical students is a GMC requirement of a medical school (General Medical Council 2009). Jennings claimed that student burnout can be attributed to a medical school culture that failed to value medical students. He called for medical schools to create learning environments that respected the integrity of students and nurtured them as professionals and people (Jennings 2009).

Promoting Empathic Professionalism
It is paradoxical that while descriptions of professionalism include humanistic values such as empathy, students gain an impression of professionalism as distancing from patients (Jeffrey 2018; Kerasidou and Horn 2016; West and Shanafelt 2007). The debate in the literature around medical professionalism mirrors much of that surrounding empathy: a lack of definition and uncertainty as to whether it can be taught or assessed (Cruess et al. 2014; Levenson et al. 2008; Rogers and Ballantyne 2010). Constructing an appropriate professional identity has become more complicated for contemporary medical students as a tension exists between a conforming culture in medical schools and increasing diversity of students (Frost and Regehr 2013; Jeffrey 2018).

Providing Time: Empathy vs Efficiency
Students express a view that empathy was inhibited by a lack of time (Eikeland et al. 2014; Nogueira-Martins et al. 2006; Ratanawongsa et al. 2005; Tavakol et al. 2012). Conversely, students claim that having adequate time helps to establish their connection with patients (Cutler

et al. 2009). While fast medicine is appropriate in emergency situations, there may be a place for slow medicine in many of the illnesses which evolve chronically (Bauer 2008). There is a need to provide time for students to reflect about their experiences (Wear et al. 2014).

Students who do spend time with patients risk being regarded as inefficient (Christakis and Feudtner 1997). A doctor should spend more time in establishing empathic relationships. Those responsible for the doctor's workload should restructure their timetables to allow for empathy to flourish (Hardy 2017).

Creating a Dialogue
Taking a history is a skilled act which requires the capacity to empathise with the patient and then to recount her story in a medical narrative (Montgomery 2006). Teaching students to be suspicious of anecdote is yet another mechanism for inhibiting the influence of emotions. The biomedical emphasis in the way students are taught to take a history is exemplified by the marginalisation of the acronym ICE; ideas, concerns and expectations. Empathy involves engaging with the patients' ideas, concerns and expectations (ICE) of their illness and its treatment (Tate 2005). Students' described how these areas of taking a history were relegated to the end of their consultation and sometimes omitted (Jeffrey 2018). This accentuated the biomedical model, relegating the psychosocial concerns to an optional add-on to the 'proper' history, resulting in further distancing from the patient.

Introducing the Humanities into the Curriculum
The arts and humanities should form part of the core curriculum in medical education. In the 1970s, medical ethics was incorporated into North American medical schools curricula in response to objections to medicine's dehumanisation of patients (Bleakley 2015b). Medical humanities, however, have failed to make a similar impact into medical school curricula and remains on the edges of medical education (Bleakley 2015b; Kumagai 2017).

Many authors pointed to the potential of the humanities to promote empathy in medical students (Batt-Rawden et al. 2013; Charon 2001; Kumagai 2017; Pedersen 2010; Shapiro et al. 2006). Bleakley suggests that incorporating the humanities into the curriculum as a core element can help to address the reductive approach of biomedicine (Bleakley

2015b). The question facing us now is not can doctors learn from the humanities? but rather how do we learn from them? Kumagai points out that one of the functions of teaching the humanities is to disturb our assumptions and prejudices and to open us to possibilities (Kumagai 2017). The humanities show us that there is no single right answer. The humanities create an ethical pause where we can step back and think deeply about other people and their lives (Kumagai 2017). They also allow students and doctors to engage a sociological perspective when thinking about the patient's story (Kumagai 2017). The arts can encourage students to see the world through the other's eyes, to empathise. The power of art lies in its ability to provoke a reaction in its audience, which depends on interpretation of the work and necessarily involves emotions (Sood and Moore 2019).

Storytelling is another effective way to learn about empathy, echoing Charon's ideas for developing narrative competence (Charon 2001; Griswold et al. 2007). The arts communicate the ambiguous, unspoken and unseen in contrast to medical communication which is focused on the factual and scientific aspects of the patient. The language of clinical medicine may distance the patient and doctor.

Empathy has a transcendent quality, in the process of caring the doctor and patient occupy a space in which they may change in fundamental ways (Kumagai 2017).

RESEARCH

Many quantitative researchers have appealed for further qualitative research into the development of medical students' empathy (Batt-Rawden et al. 2013; Pedersen 2010). The focus of future research in clinical empathy should explore empathy as a two-way relationship with the patient, rather than being an attribute of the student or doctor. It seems that rather than repeating quantitative measurements of empathy it would be more productive to carry out further longitudinal phenomenological research to explore the effects of the explicit and hidden curricula (Jeffrey 2018). There is a need to research the views of students in medical schools, their medical educators and patients.

Future research should be directed at understanding the components of empathy that improve patient satisfaction, clinical outcomes and physician well-being (Kiosses et al. 2016; Stepien and Baernstein 2006).

Such understanding might allow teachers to target their interventions on specific dimensions of empathy (Stepien and Baernstein 2006).

In Western society, the positivist ideas of science prevail to an extent that science is assumed to represent uninfluenced reality beyond interpretation (Montgomery 2006). Perhaps it is not surprising then that medicine distrusts anecdotes. Yet, paradoxically, clinical medicine begins with a patient's story. Phenomenological research and clinical medicine rely both on a negotiation, between the individual story and the background evidence, on interpretation and reflexivity (Hopkins and Dudley-Evans 1988; Montgomery 2006).

One of the inevitable limitations of research in the social sciences is that it can never be possible to know fully what another person is thinking and feeling. However, the fact that a perfect understanding is not possible does not invalidate the knowledge generated by thorough, sensitive qualitative research (Finlay and Gough 2008).

Conclusion

Embedding empathy into clinical practice begins by clarifying a relational view of empathy which includes emotions. The context of the patient-doctor relationship is critical, empathy-based ethics requires presence, time, a pause for reflection and continuity of care. The patient's experience of their illness needs to be at the heart of the consultation, the doctor adopting a phenomenological approach. In this way, a balance can be reached between biomedical and psychosocial aspects of the patient's illness.

Embedding the empathy-based ethical framework into medical undergraduate curriculum reinforces the importance of empathy. The humanities provide a rich source of learning around empathy-based ethics and need to be integral to the students' learning throughout the curriculum, not simply as an add-on module.

Research on empathy in medicine has been largely involved with attempts to measure empathy in students and doctors. What is now needed are longitudinal qualitative studies, involving clinicians, patients, students and their teachers, to explore the factors which influence empathy.

The final chapter looks to the future and the challenges faced in implementing such changes in order to humanise medical practice and education.

REFERENCES

Ahrweiler, F., Neumann, M., Goldblatt, H., Hahn, E. G., & Scheffer, C. (2014). Determinants of physician empathy during medical education: Hypothetical conclusions from an exploratory qualitative survey of practicing physicians. *BMC Medical Education, 14,* 122–134. https://doi.org/10.1186/1472-6920-14-122.

Ballatt, J., & Campling, P. (2011). *Intelligent kindness*. London: RCPsych Publications.

Batt-Rawden, S., Chisolm, M. S., Anton, B., & Flickinger, T. E. (2013). Teaching empathy to medical students: An updated, systematic review. *Academic Medicine, 88*(8), 1171–1177.

Bauer, J. L. (2008). Slow Medicine. *The Journal of Alternative and Complementary Medicine, 14,* 891–892.

Bayne, H. B. (2011). Training medical students in empathic communication. *The Journal for Specialists in Group Work, 36*(4), 316–329.

Bleakley, A. (2015b). When I say ... the medical humanities in education. *Medical Education, 49,* 959–960.

Bleakley, A., & Bligh, J. (2008). Students learning from patients: Let's get real in medical education. *Advances in Health Sciences Education, 13*(1), 89–107.

Branch, W. T. (2010). The road to professionalism: Reflective practice and reflective learning. *Patient Education and Counseling, 80*(3), 327–332.

Brandl, K., Schneid, S. D., Smith, S., Winegarden, B., Mandel, J., & Kelly, C. J. (2017). Small group activities within academic communities improve the connectedness of students and faculty. *Medical Teacher,* 1–7.

Brazeau, C., Schroeder, R., Rovi, S., & Boyd, L. (2010). Relationships between medical student burnout, empathy, and professionalism climate. *Academic Medicine, 85*(10), 33–36.

Cacioppo, J. T., Hawkley, L. C., Norman, G. J., & Berntson, G. G. (2011). Social isolation. *Annals of the New York Academy of Sciences, 1231*(1), 17–22.

Carel, H. (2016). *The phenomenology of illness*. Oxford: Oxford University Press.

Charon, R. (2001). Narrative medicine—A model for empathy, reflection, profession, and trust. *JAMA, 286*(15), 1897–1902. https://doi.org/10.1001/jama.286.15.1897.

Chen, D., Lew, R., Hershman, W., & Orlander, J. (2007). A cross-sectional measurement of medical student empathy. *Journal of General Internal Medicine, 22*(10), 1434–1438. https://doi.org/10.1007/s11606-007-0298-x.

Christakis, D., & Feudtner, C. (1997). Temporary matters: The ethical consequences of transient social relationships in medical training. *JAMA, 278*(9), 739–743.

Cleland, J. (2015). Exploring versus measuring: Considering the fundamental differences between qualitative and quantitative research. In J. Cleland & S.

Durning (Eds.), *Researching medical education*. London: John Wiley & Sons Ltd.

Cohen, L. G., & Sherif, Y. A. (2014). Twelve tips on teaching and learning humanism in medical education. *Medical Teacher, 36*(8), 680–684.

Coulehan, J. L. (1995). Tenderness and steadiness: Emotions in medical practice. *Literature and Medicine, 14*(2), 222–236.

Cruess, R. L., Cruess, S. R., Boudreau, J. D., Snell, L., & Steinert, Y. (2014). Reframing medical education to support professional identity formation. *Academic Medicine, 89*(11), 1446–1451.

Cutler, J., Harding, K., Mozian, S., Wright, L. L., Pica, A. G., Masters, S., et al. (2009). Discrediting the notion "working with 'crazies' will make you 'crazy'": Addressing stigma and enhancing empathy in medical student education. *Advances in Health Sciences Education, 14*(4), 487–502. https://doi.org/10.1007/s10459-008-9132-4.

Davis, C. M. (1990). What is empathy, and can empathy be taught? *Physical Therapy, 70*(11), 707–711.

Decety, J., & Meyer, M. (2008). From emotion resonance to empathic understanding: A social developmental neuroscience account. *Development and Psychopathology, 20*(4), 1053–1080.

Dyrbye, L. N., Thomas, M. R., & Shanafelt, T. D. (2005). Medical student distress: Causes, consequences and proposed solutions. *Mayo Clinic Proceedings, 80*(12), 1613–1622.

Egnew, T. R., & Wilson, H. J. (2010). Faculty and medical students' perceptions of teaching and learning about the doctor–patient relationship. *Patient Education and Counseling, 79*(2), 199–206.

Eikeland, H. L., Ornes, K., Finset, A., & Pedersen, R. (2014). The physician's role and empathy—A qualitative study of third year medical students. *BMC Medical Education, 14,* 165–173. https://doi.org/10.1186/1472-6920-14-165.

Ekman, E., & Halpern, J. (2015). Professional distress and meaning in health care: Why professional empathy can help. *Social Work in Health Care, 54*(7), 633–650.

Elder, A., & Verghese, A. (2015). Bedside matters-putting the patient at the centre of teaching and learning. *Royal College of Physicians of Edinburgh, 45*(3), 186–187.

Engel, G. L. (1977). The need of a new medical model: A challenge for biomedicine. *Science, 196,* 129–136.

Finlay, L. (2013). Unfolding the phenomenological research process: Iterative stages of "seeing a fresh". *Journal of Humanistic Psychology, 53*(2), 172–201.

Finlay, L., & Gough, B. (2008). *Reflexivity: A practical guide for researchers in health and social sciences*. Chichester: John Wiley & Sons.

Foster, W., & Freeman, E. (2008). Poetry in general practice education: Perceptions of learners. *Family Practice, 25*(4), 294–303.

Frost, H. D., & Regehr, G. (2013). "I am a doctor": Negotiating the discourses of standardization and diversity in professional identity construction. *Academic Medicine, 88*(10), 1570–1577.

General Medical Council. (2009). *Tomorrow's doctors: Outcomes and standards for undergraduate medical education.* Retrieved from London.

General Medical Council. (2019). *The state of medical education and practice in the UK.* Retrieved from https://www.gmc-uk.org/-/media/documents/somep-2019—executive-summary_pdf-81141889.pdf?la=en&hash=B61311 F70D2DAA8FF8FEB8BA0B44805AFB713C5A.

Genn, J. (2001). AMEE Medical Education Guide No. 23 (Part 1): Curriculum, environment, climate, quality and change in medical education—A unifying perspective. *Medical Teacher, 23*(4), 337–344.

George, S., & Gerada, C. (2019). Stressed GPs: A call for action. *British Journal of General Practice, 69*, 116–117.

Georgi, E., Petermann, F., & Schipper, M. (2014). Are empathic abilities learnable? Implications for social neuroscientific research from psychometric assessments. *Social Neuroscience, 9*(1), 74–81. https://doi.org/10.1080/174 70919.2013.855253.

Griswold, K., Zayas, L., Kernan, J. B., & Wagner, C. M. (2007). Cultural awareness through medical student and refugee patient encounters. *Journal of Immigrant and Minority Health, 9*(1), 55–60.

Hafferty, F. W. (1998). Beyond curriculum reform: Confronting medicine's hidden curriculum. *Academic Medicine, 73*(4), 403–407.

Halpern, J. (2001). *From detached concern to empathy: Humanizing medical practice.* Oxford: Oxford University Press.

Hardy, C. (2017). Empathizing with patients: The role of interaction and narratives in providing better patient care. *Medicine, Healthcare and Philosophy, 20,* 237–248.

Hooker, C. (2015). Understanding empathy: Why phenomenology and hermeneutics can help medical education and practice. *Medicine, Health Care and Philosophy, 18*(4), 541–552.

Hopkins, A., & Dudley-Evans, T. (1988). A genre-based investigation of the discussion sections in articles and dissertations. *English for Specific Purposes, 7*(2), 113–121.

Imo, U. O. (2017). Burnout and psychiatric morbidity among doctors in the UK: A systematic literature review of prevalence and associated factors. *BJPsych Bulletin, 41,* 197–204.

Janssen, A. L., & MacLeod, R. D. (2010). What can people approaching death teach us about how to care? *Patient Education and Counseling, 81*(2), 251–256. https://doi.org/10.1016/j.pec.2010.02.009.

Janssen, A. L., Macleod, R. D., & Walker, S. T. (2008). Recognition, reflection, and role models: Critical elements in education about care in medicine. *Palliative & Supportive Care, 6*(4), 389–395. https://doi.org/10.1017/s14 78951508000618.

Jeffrey, D. (2014). *Medical mentoring: Supporting students, doctors in training and general practitioners.* London: Royal College of General Practitioners.

Jeffrey, D. (2016a). Clarifying empathy: The first step to more humane clinical care. *British Journal of General Practice, 66,* 101–102.

Jeffrey, D. (2017). Communicating with a human voice: Developing a relational model of empathy. *Journal of the Royal College of Physicians of Edinburgh, 47*(3), 267.

Jeffrey, D. (2018). *Exploring empathy with medical students: A qualitative longitudinal phenomenological study.* (PhD), University of Edinburgh. Retrieved from https://www.pure.ed.ac.uk/admin/editor/dk/atira/pure/api/sha red/model/base_uk/studentthesis/editor/studentthesiseditor.xhtml?id=592 49782. Accessed 6 June 2018.

Jeffrey, D., & Downie, R. (2016). Empathy-Can it be taught? *Journal of the Royal College of Physicians of Edinburgh, 46,* 107–112.

Jennings, M. (2009). Medical student burnout: Interdisciplinary exploration and analysis. *Journal of Medical Humanities, 30*(4), 253–269.

Karnieli-Miller, O., Vu, T. R., Frankel, R. M., Holtman, M. C., Clyman, S. G., Hui, S. L., et al. (2011). Which experiences in the hidden curriculum teach students about professionalism? *Academic Medicine, 86*(3), 369–377. https://doi.org/10.1097/ACM.0b013e3182087d15.

Kelm, Z., Womer, J., Walter, J., & Feudtner, C. (2014). Interventions to cultivate physician empathy: A systematic review. *BMC Medical Education, 14*(1), 219–230.

Kerasidou, A., & Horn, R. (2016). Making space for empathy: supporting doctors in the emotional labour of clinical care. *BMC Medical Ethics, 17*(1), 8–13.

Kinman, G., & Teoh, K. (2018). *What could make a difference to the mental health of UK doctors? A review of the research evidence.* Retrieved from https://eprints.bbk.ac.uk/24540/1/2018.%20LTF%20SOM%20Mental% 20health%20of%20UK%20doctors.pdf.

Kiosses, V. N., Karathanos, V. T., & Tatsioni, A. (2016). Empathy promoting interventions for health professionals: A systematic review of RCTs. *Journal of Compassionate Health Care, 3*(1), 7–29.

Kozlowski, D., Hutchinson, M., Hurley, J., Rowley, J., & Sutherland, J. (2017). The role of emotion in clinical decision making: An integrative literature review. *BMC Medical Education, 17*(1), 255–268.

Kumagai, A. K. (2017). Beyond "Dr. Feel-Good": A role for the humanities in medical education. *Academic Medicine, 92,* 1659–1660.

Lempp, H., & Seale, C. (2004). The hidden curriculum in undergraduate medical education: Qualitative study of medical students' perceptions of teaching. *BMJ, 329*(7469), 770–773.

Levenson, R., Dewar, S., & Shepherd, S. (2008). *Understanding doctors.* Retrieved from London.

Lutz, G., Scheffer, C., Edelhaeuser, F., Tauschel, D., & Neumann, M. (2013). A reflective practice intervention for professional development, reduced stress and improved patient care—A qualitative developmental evaluation. *Patient Education and Counseling, 92*(3), 337–345.

Marcum, J. A. (2013). The role of empathy and wisdom in Medical Practice and Pedagogy: Confronting the Hidden Curriculum. *Journal of Biomedical Education, 2013,* 1–8.

Marshall, R., & Bleakley, A. (2009). The death of hector: Pity in Homer, empathy in medical education. *Medical Humanities, 35*(1), 7–12. https://doi.org/10.1136/jmh.2008.001081.

Maxwell, B. (2008). *Professional ethics education: Studies in compassionate empathy.* New York: Springer.

Maxwell, B., & Racine, E. (2010). Should empathic development be a priority in biomedical ethics teaching? A critical perspective. *Cambridge Quarterly of Healthcare Ethics, 19*(4), 433–445. https://doi.org/10.1017/s0963180110000320.

Mayer, J. D., Salovey, P., & Caruso, D. R. (2008). Emotional intelligence: New ability or eclectic traits? *American Psychologist, 63*(6), 503–517.

Meier, D. E., Back, A., & Morrison, R. (2001). The inner life of physicians and care of the seriously ill. *JAMA, 286*(23), 3007–3014.

Monrouxe, L. V., & Rees, C. E. (2012). "It's just a clash of cultures": Emotional talk within medical students' narratives of professionalism dilemmas. *Advances in Health Sciences Education, 17*(5), 671–701.

Monrouxe, L. V., Rees, C. E., Endacott, R., & Ternan, E. (2014). 'Even now it makes me angry': Health care students' professionalism dilemma narratives. *Medical Education, 48*(5), 502–517.

Monrouxe, L. V., Rees, C. E., & Hu, W. (2011). Differences in medical students' explicit discourses of professionalism: Acting, representing, becoming. *Medical Education, 45*(6), 585–602.

Montgomery, K. (2006). *How doctors think: Clinical judgment and the practice of medicine.* Oxford: Oxford University Press.

Nogueira-Martins, M. C. F., Nogueira-Martins, L. A., & Turato, E. R. (2006). Medical students' perceptions of their learning about the doctor-patient relationship: A qualitative study. *Medical Education, 40*(4), 322–328. https://doi.org/10.1111/j.1365-2929.2006.02411.x.

Ozbay, F., Johnson, D. C., Dimoulas, E., Morgan, C., III, Charney, D., & Southwick, S. (2007). Social support and resilience to stress: From neurobiology to clinical practice. *Psychiatry, 4*(5), 35.

Paro, H. M. S., Silveira, P. S. P., Perotta, B., Gannam, S., Enns, S. C., Giaxa, R. R. B., et al. (2014). Empathy among medical students: Is there a relation with quality of life and burnout? *PLoS ONE, 9*(4), e94133–e94133. https://doi.org/10.1371/journal.pone.0094133.

Passi, V., Johnson, S., Peile, E., Wright, S., Hafferty, F., & Johnson, N. (2013). Doctor role modelling in medical education: BEME Guide No. 27. *Medical Teacher, 35*(9), e1422–e1436.

Pedersen, R. (2009). Empirical research on empathy in medicine-A critical review. *Patient Education and Counseling, 76*(3), 307–322. https://doi.org/10.1016/j.pec.2009.06.012.

Pedersen, R. (2010). Empathy development in medical education—A critical review. *Medical Teacher, 32*(7), 593–600. https://doi.org/10.3109/014215 90903544702.

Perrella, A. (2016). Fool me once: The illusion of empathy in interactions with standardized patients. *Medical Teacher, 38*(12), 1285–1287.

Ramesh, A. (2013). A call for reflection: Medical student driven effort to foster empathy and compassion. *Medical Teacher, 35*(1), 69–70. https://doi.org/10.3109/0142159x.2012.731109.

Ratanawongsa, N., Teherani, A., & Hauer, K. E. (2005). Third-year medical students' experiences with dying patients during the internal medicine clerkship: A qualitative study of the informal curriculum. *Academic Medicine, 80*(7), 641–647.

Reblin, M., & Uchino, B. N. (2008). Social and emotional support and its implication for health. *Current Opinion in Psychiatry, 21*(2), 201–205.

Rees, C. E., & Monrouxe, L. V. (2011). "A morning since eight of just pure grill": A multischool qualitative study of student abuse. *Academic Medicine, 86*(11), 1374–1382.

Rees, C. E., Monrouxe, L. V., & McDonald, L. A. (2013). Narrative, emotion and action: Analysing 'most memorable'professionalism dilemmas. *Medical Education, 47*(1), 80–96.

Rogers, W., & Ballantyne, A. (2010). Towards a practical definition of professional behaviour. *Journal of Medical Ethics, 36*(4), 250–254.

Sanchez-Reilly, S., Morrison, L. J., Carey, E., Bernacki, R., O'Neill, L., Kapo, J., et al. (2013). Caring for oneself to care for others: Physicians and their self-care. *The Journal of Supportive Oncology, 11*(2), 75–81.

Schön, D. A. (1987). *Educating the reflective practitioner: Toward a new design for teaching and learning in the professions.* San Francisco: Jossey-Bass.

Shanafelt, T., West, C., Zhao, X. H., Novotny, P., Kolars, J., Habermann, T., et al. (2005). Relationship between increased personal well-being and enhanced empathy among internal medicine residents. *Journal of General Internal Medicine, 20*(7), 559–564. https://doi.org/10.1111/j.1365-1497. 2005.0108.x.

Shapiro, J. (2008). Walking a mile in their patients' shoes: Empathy and othering in medical students' education. *Philosophy, Ethics, and Humanities in Medicine, 3,* 10–21.

Shapiro, J. (2012). The paradox of teaching empathy. In Medical Students In & J. Decety (Eds.), *Empathy: From bench to bedside.* Cambridge, MA: MIT Press.

Shapiro, J., Rucker, L., & Robitshek, D. (2006). Teaching the art of doctoring: An innovative medical student elective. *Medical Teacher, 28*(1), 30–35.

Sheikh, H., Carpenter, J., & Wee, J. (2013). Medical student reporting of factors affecting pre-clerkship changes in empathy: A qualitative study. *Canadian Medical Education Journal, 4*(1), e26–e34.

Smith, J. A., Flowers, P., & Larkin, M. (2009). *Interpretative phenomenological analysis: Theory, method and research.* London: Sage.

Sood, M., & Moore, J. (2019). Empathy, emotional attachment, and the end. *British Journal of General Practice* (March), 132. https://doi.org/10.3399/ bjgp19X701525.

Stepien, K. A., & Baernstein, A. (2006). Educating for empathy—A review. *Journal of General Internal Medicine, 21*(5), 524–530. https://doi.org/10. 1111/j.1525-1497.2006.00443.x.

Tate, P. (2005). Ideas, concerns and expectations. *Medicine, 33*(2), 26–27.

Tavakol, S., Dennick, R., & Tavakol, M. (2012). Medical students' understanding of empathy: A phenomenological study. *Medical Education, 46*(7), 306–316. https://doi.org/10.1111/j.1365-2923.2012.04305.x.

Timm, A. (2014). 'It would not be tolerated in any other profession except medicine': Survey reporting on undergraduates' exposure to bullying and harassment in their first placement year. *BMJ Open, 4*(7), e005140. Retrieved from http://dx.doi.org/10.1136/bmjopen-2014-005140 and https://doi. org/10.1136/bmjopen-2014-005140.

Underman, K. (2015). Playing doctor: Simulation in medical school as affective practice. *Social Science and Medicine, 136,* 180–188.

Underman, K., & Hirshfield, L. E. (2016). Detached concern?: Emotional socialization in twenty-first century medical education. *Social Science and Medicine, 160,* 94–101.

Vagle, M. D. (2010). Re-framing Schön's call for a phenomenology of practice: A post-intentional approach. *Reflective Practice, 11*(3), 393–407.

Van Manen, M. (2016). *Researching lived experience: Human science for an action sensitive pedagogy.* London: Routledge.

Wear, D., & Varley, J. D. (2008). Rituals of verification: The role of simulation in developing and evaluating empathic communication. *Patient Education and Counseling, 71*(2), 153–156.

Wear, D., Zarconi, J., Kumagai, A., & Cole-Kelly, K. (2014). Slow medical education. *Academic Medicine, 90,* 289–293.

West, M., & Coia, D. (2019). *Caring for doctors caring for patients.* Retrieved from http://www.rcpe.ac.uk/sites/default/files/caring_for_doctors.pdf.

West, C. P., & Shanafelt, T. D. (2007). The influence of personal and environmental factors on professionalism in medical education. *BMC Medical Education, 7*(1), 29–38.

Winseman, J., Malik, A., Morison, J., & Balkoski, V. (2009). Students' views on factors affecting empathy in medical education. *Academic Psychiatry, 33*(6), 484–491.

Woloschuk, W., Harasym, P. H., & Temple, W. (2004). Attitude change during medical school: A cohort study. *Medical Education, 38*(5), 522–534.

Wright, S. M., Kern, D. E., Kolodner, K., Howard, D. M., & Brancati, F. L. (1998). Attributes of excellent attending-physician role models. *New England Journal of Medicine, 339*(27), 1986–1993.

CHAPTER 10

The Future: Empathy-Based Ethics (EBE) and Humane Medical Practice

Abstract The ethical requirement for humanity in health care is apparent, the challenge is to integrate the empathy-based ethics approach into everyday clinical practice. Adopting an empathy-based ethics would ensure that the patient-doctor relationship regains its core value. Physicians need a feeling of personal responsibility for the care of the patient, which is compatible with working in a multidisciplinary team. Changes in the culture of the NHS, clinical practice and education are explored. There is a need to move away from the polarity between the biomedical and psychosocial aspects of care. There is a need to shift from an authority-led hierarchy that is doctor-centred to a patient-centred approach fostering humane interactions in medicine and integration of the humanities into education. Empathy-based ethics extends the ethical importance of empathy from a desirable moral disposition in a doctor to a capacity which is fundamental to ethical functioning.

Keywords Empathy-based ethics · Patient-doctor relationship · Organisational culture · Medical humanities · Medical education

© The Author(s), under exclusive license to Springer Nature Switzerland AG 2020
D. I. Jeffrey, *Empathy-Based Ethics*,
https://doi.org/10.1007/978-3-030-64804-6_10

INTRODUCTION

The preceding chapters have reviewed how a lack of empathy contributed to the lack of humane care of patients, highlighted in the Francis Report(Francis 2013). Having identified the causes of medical dehumanisation and clarified a relational concept of empathy, I have described a fresh clinical empathy-based ethical approach to humanising medical practice. An empathy-based approach to medical ethics which can be embedded in clinical practice, medical education and research has evolved, the challenges involved in implementing this approach are now discussed.

The empathy-based ethics (EBE) approach responds to the current culture of stress, patient dissatisfaction and the empathy gap in health care (Derksen et al. 2020; Shanafelt et al. 2005). At the heart of the EBE approach is the patient-doctor relationship. Empathy-based ethics embraces a broad concept of empathy which includes emotions and the motivation to act in the best interests of the individual patient. Reflection and self-awareness are fostered in mentoring relationships, generating optimal outcomes from moral deliberation.

Empathy-based ethics draws on a variety of philosophical perspectives. Phenomenology focuses on interpreting the patient's experience of their illness from their point of view. Virtue ethics, especially sympathy, kindness generosity and humility determine the character of the good doctor. Care ethics considers the welfare of both the patient and the doctor in the context of their relationship.

Levinas asserts that when two people meet each other both of them put a value on their meeting, creating a relationship, a space for a narrative, which allows them to understand each other better (Levinas 2006). At the heart of the patient-doctor relationship is the consultation; a process of listening, telling, reflection, interpretation and mutual understanding. During this reciprocal process of mutual respect, the doctor comes to learn more about the patient and the patient more about the doctor. Patients look to their doctor to affirm that they matter, seeking empathic concern, attentiveness, respectful dialogue and commitment (Chochinov 2007; Warmington 2012). Attentiveness involves not only thinking of the other person and being present for them but also communicating concern for their care (Derksen et al. 2020; Klaver & Baart 2016).The empathy-based approach gives the doctor a detailed view of the patient's ideas, concerns, assumptions, values and hopes in the context of their social situation.

Empathy-based ethics sees each individual as having human dignity and being of equal worth (Nussbaum 2013). There are inevitable power differences in the patient-doctor relationship but an empathic approach is committed to reducing these as much as possible, enabling the patient to raise difficult emotional concerns in a true dialogue(Derksen et al. 2020). Empathy-based ethics leads to a more humane form of practice, as the patient and the doctor are seen as individuals within a context. Ricoeur argued that despite the differences which separate us from one another we are inevitably bound in a quest for mutual recognition and understanding (Ricoeur 1992). Selfhood and otherness cannot be separated, once we are able to see oneself as another implies being able to see another as oneself. In this manner, the suffering of others becomes our suffering (Shapiro 2008).

The ethical requirement for humanity in health care is apparent, the challenge is to integrate the empathy-based ethics approach into everyday clinical practice (Gillon 2013). In the 1990s, Weatherall warned of the inhumanity of medicine and suggested that we seem to be becoming "a profession of uncaring technocrats" (Weatherall 1994). Despite repeated calls to restore the human face of medicine little has changed (Gillon 2013). The challenge of humanising medical practice has been debated for half a century (Konner 1987).

Despite arguing for the centrality of empathy in the patient-doctor relationship over many years and developing communication skill courses, there has not been a dramatic shift towards humane practice (Jeffrey 2019; Shapiro 2008). Modern medicine is mediated by technology, instead of touching the patient, scans are substituted for personal closeness. Understanding becomes diagnosis and prognosis, assistance becomes treatment (Shapiro 2008). The mechanistic view that science imposes on suffering risks reducing a patient to a disease, an object. Transforming patients into objects or tasks rather than human beings is a way of avoiding unscientific emotional entanglement and fosters the "othering" of the patient (Shapiro 2008). In spite of efforts to empathise as a way of drawing close to the patient, empathy does not accord with the prevailing biomedical model, but instead it seems like something to be added to the consultation, time permitting (Jeffrey 2018). Biomedical knowledge is appropriate in certain situations but we need to acknowledge there may be equivalent sources of other knowledge that may be more relevant in determining how to be in relationship with a patient. Biomedical knowledge cannot produce empathy (Shapiro 2008). Change in the culture of the NHS, clinical practice, education and research are explored in this concluding chapter.

Implementing EBE in Clinical Practice

Patient-Doctor Relationship

Placing a greater emphasis on personalised care strengthens the patient-doctor relationship. Amongst the challenges facing doctors aiming to deliver such care are a lack of time and providing continuity of care. Clinical practice now depends on a collaborative team approach but even a simple introduction and pause to listen to the patient's concerns can humanise care (Granger 2013). By giving the patient undivided attention the doctor can convey their interest and concern with the patient's experience of their illness. How patients perceive themselves to be seen by doctors is a significant mediator of their dignity (Chochinov 2007). Chochinov suggests that the more that doctors are able to affirm the patient's value, seeing them as unique individuals, the more their sense of dignity will be retained (Chochinov 2007). Physicians need a feeling of personal responsibility for the care of the patient, which is compatible with working in a multidisciplinary team (Haque and Waytz 2012).

The patient-doctor relationship based on empathy is one of mutual trust, respect and shared decision-making. Empathy reduces the power differences between doctor and patient a process which can be helped by promoting doctor-patient similarity, by encouraging racial, ethnic, and gender diversity in physician populations to match patient demographics, a challenge for recruitment (Haque and Waytz 2012).

Patients should not be labelled as their disease, instead, their shared humanity should be acknowledged. Patients need to be identified in a more personal manner than simply checking their identity and date of birth on a wristband. Personal identification of the patient would serve to remind doctors of their shared humanity. It is accepted that empathy improves patient outcomes, reduces medical errors and reduces burnout, yet doctors need a favourable organisational culture to develop empathic relationships with patients (Howick and Rees 2017).

Adopting an empathy-based ethical approach at the heart of clinical practice would ensure that the patient-doctor relationship regains its core value. Empathy depends upon the connection between the doctor and patient, an engagement which requires both physical and psychological closeness. Hospital patients are dressed in skimpy gowns which barely cover private parts. They are required to use bedpans and commodes behind a screen yet audible to other members of the ward, a dehumanising lack of privacy. Clothing which facilitates physical examination need not also humiliate people who are at their most vulnerable, allowing observers to morally disengage from them. The psychological and moral distance created by technology in medical settings also facilitates moral disengagement and consequent dehumanisation (Haque and Waytz 2012). Much of the care that doctors automatically provide in face-to-face medical interactions diminishes when technology is introduced to diagnosis and treatment (Haque and Waytz 2012).

Organisational Culture

Gillon suggests that we need to move away from the polarity between the biomedical and psychosocial aspects of care (Gillon 2013). He calls the scientific bias 'biomedical machismo' and argues for abolishing this approach (Gillon 2013). He identifies the importance of changing the attitudes of some powerful individuals, holding biomedical machismo, who lead Trusts, hospitals, universities and affect the ethos of the group they influence (Gillon 2013).

The need for change extends beyond individual doctors to involve the institutional culture of clinical practice and medical education. There is a need to shift from an authority-led hierarchy that is doctor-centred to a patient-centred approach. The organisational culture often adopts an approach which infers "this is the way we do things here".

There is a need to emphasise the importance of humanity in the delivery of health and social care (Gillon 2013). The King's Fund Point of Care programme focused on Empathy and Compassion, work which continue in The Point of Care Foundation (Point of Care Foundation 2013; The King's Fund 2013). The Point of Care Foundation in the UK, have adopted Schwartz Center Rounds, developed in the USA, which bring together hospital staff to discuss emotional and psychological care of patients in a group setting (Goodrich 2012). These have increased empathy, peer support, reflection, improved communication with patients and improved staff well-being (Maben et al. 2017; Taylor et al. 2018).

Recently, there have been initiatives in the UK to enhance empathy in healthcare settings as a response to the perceived need to humanise medical care (Shea & Lionis, 2014). One example is the online

Connecting, Assessing, Responding and Empowering (CARE) approach developed at the University of Glasgow to enhance empathy in primary care staff (Bikker et al. 2012; Fitzgerald et al. 2014).

The NHS Constitution emphasises themes of compassion, dignity and respect (The Department of Health and Social Care 2015). Gillon suggests setting up a Humanity Task force to oversee practice and ensure these values are integrated into everyday care (Gillon 2013). This is not to decry biomedical skills but simply to balance these with humanity. Gillon makes a plea for healthcare workers to have time with patients. Each health care worker should ask themselves, 'Is my practice humane?' (Gillon 2013).

Berwick has named the present time as Era 3 medicine; Era 1 being a time doctors judged their own work, while Era 2, focused on accountability and targets. Era 3 is to be the 'moral era' where we hear the voices of the people served, moving on from asking "what's the matter with you?" to "what matters to you?" (Berwick 2016).

MEDICAL UNDERGRADUATE EDUCATION

It has been argued that medical school education is a process of assimilation into a culture of objectivity (Gordon 1995). There have been changes in medical undergraduate curricula, as a result of initiatives such as the GMC's publication, *Tomorrow's Doctors*, which have led to an outcome-based approach to undergraduate medical education (General Medical Council 2009). One consequence of these changes is that the professional socialisation of medical students is now more defined (Underman and Hirshfield 2016).There have also been demographic changes in the medical student population with more female students and a racially diverse student community (Underman and Hirshfield 2016).These welcome developments have occurred against a background of changes in clinical practice such as: evidence-based medicine, increasing patient consumerism and a sophisticated technology which stresses a biomedical view of medical practice (Howick and Rees 2017; Montgomery 2006; Underman and Hirshfield 2016).

Haslam suggests that empathy, which enhances the doctor-patient relationship, might form a selection criteria for entry to medical school (Haslam 2007). Bleakley identifies inequality in power as a factor which dehumanises medicine, for example, bedside teaching can involve the humiliation of students (Bleakley 2015). He suggests a need to democratise humane interactions in medicine and integration of the humanities into education (Bleakley 2015). The humanities can change doctors who prioritise a smart diagnosis over a patient's feelings, by increasing moral sensibility to ways of behaving. 70% of medical errors are grounded in communication problems between doctors and their colleagues or patients (Schafer et al. 1994). However, it is clear that communication skills training is failing to humanise medicine (Bleakley 2015). Medical education should also incorporate practices that emphasise the common humanity students share with patients.

Students continue to have negative perceptions about sociology in their undergraduate education (Brooks et al. 2016). The biomedical model remains deeply entrenched within medical practice and medical education, acting as a barrier to students' acceptance of sociology as an integral part of their studies (Brooks et al. 2016). A growing interest in social constructivist theories and qualitative research presents an opportunity for sociologists to challenge organisational cultures which influence students' perceptions (Jeffrey 2018).

Moral development involves not only moral reasoning but includes moral motivation, moral character and moral sensitivity; empathy is involved in each of these dimensions (Maxwell 2008). Educationalists have questioned how to extend ethics teaching beyond skills of moral reasoning. The most frequent suggestion has been to provide support for empathic relationships (Maxwell 2008). The aim of ethics education is to promote the performance of moral actions. Empathy-based ethics extends the ethical importance of empathy from a desirable moral disposition in a doctor to a capacity which is fundamental to ethical functioning (Maxwell 2008).

Educational approaches and a learning culture are needed that can help students learn from their emotions (Shapiro 2008). Role models who exhibit vulnerability can help students to recognise and explore difficult conversations rather than distancing themselves from patients. They need to acknowledge the incomplete nature of their understanding yet willingness to share in the patient's suffering (Shapiro 2008). To see all humanity as suffering and struggling demands humility, creates a bond and emphasises the need to treat the patient with kindness (Shapiro 2008). By focusing on the patient's subjective experience of the disease, the patient becomes the teacher. Teaching relational empathy-based ethics explores the moral implications of how to be in relation to another. It involves reflective practice with a mentor or in a small group. The relegation of emotions as unsafe in clinical training has contributed to a lack of a study of the humanities in medical education and so further diminished their visibility in training (McNaughton 2013). Literature can extend concern for others by developing imaginative reflective practice (Nussbaum 2003). Too often these activities are on the fringes of medical education but should be central to medicine culture change, the basic premises of medical education need to be humanised (Shapiro 2008).

A study of medical students' views on professionalism revealed that students who had delayed contact with patients had a restricted view of professionalism, focused on dressing and acting as a professional (Monrouxe et al. 2011). However, those who experienced early patient contact developed a more sophisticated concept of professionalism (Monrouxe et al. 2011). The authors concluded that becoming a professional was an interpersonal and complex activity which needed to be nurtured in the formal curriculum (Monrouxe et al. 2011).

MEDICAL EDUCATION RESEARCH

The question has been raised as to whether medical education research should be constructed as a medical or social science (Monrouxe and Rees 2009). Authors have argued that theories of social construction, the investigation of people's understanding of the world and how these understandings affect them, could enrich medical education research (Hirshfield and Underman 2017; Underman and Hirshfield 2016). Phenomenology is one type of constructivist research which could be employed to explore questions of racial and gender differences in empathy, the reported variation in empathy in different medical specialities and the organisational culture of a hospital or medical school (Hirshfield & Underman, 2017). Such research has the potential to inform theory, improve practice and change policy (Monrouxe and Rees 2009).

CONCLUSIONS

Employing an empathy-based approach to medical ethics in clinical practice and medical education offers a way of redressing the imbalance between biomedical and psychosocial care and humanising patient care. There needs to be a change in the organisational culture of the NHS and in universities to enhance empathic relationships between patients and doctors. The empathy-based approach to ethics developed in this book can permeate future medical education, clinical practice and research to improve the quality of the patient-doctor relationship and so enhance care.

REFERENCES

Berwick, D. M. (2016). Era 3 for medicine and health care. *JAMA, 315*(13), 1329–1330.

Bikker, A. P., Mercer, S. W., & Cotton, P. (2012). Connecting, Assessing, Responding and Empowering (CARE): A universal approach to person-centred, empathic healthcare encounters. *Education for Primary Care, 23,* 454–457.

Bleakley, A. (2015). *Medical education: How the medical humanities can shape better doctors.* London: Routledge.

Brooks, L., Collett, T., & Forrest, S. (2016). *It's just common sense! Why do negative perceptions of sociology teaching in medical education persist and is there any change in sight?*

Chochinov, H. (2007). Dignity and the essence of medicine: The A, B, C, and D of dignity conserving care. *BMJ, 335,* 184–187.

Derksen, F. A. W. M., Hartman, T. O., & Lagro-Janssen,T. (2020). The human encounter, attention, and equality: The value of doctor–patient contact. *British Journal of General Practice, 70,* 254–255.

Fitzgerald, N. M., Heywood, S., Bikker, A. P., & Mercer, S. W. (2014). Enhancing empathy in healthcare: Mixed-method evaluation of a pilot project implementing the CARE Approach in primary and community care settings in Scotland. *Journal of Compassionate Health Care, 1*(1), 1.

Francis, R. (2013). *Report of the mid staffordshire NHS foundation trust public inquiry: Executive summary.* London: HMSO.

General Medical Council. (2009). *Tomorrow's doctors: Outcomes and standards for undergraduate medical education.* Retrieved from London.

Gillon, R. (2013). Restoring humanity in health and social care–Some suggestions. *Clinical Ethics, 8*(4), 105–110.

Goodrich, J. (2012). Supporting hospital staff to provide compassionate care: Do Schwartz Center Rounds work in English hospitals? *Journal of the Royal Society of Medicine, 105*(3), 117–122.

Gordon, L. (1995). Mental health of medical students: The culture of objectivity in medicine. *The Pharos of Alpha Omega Alpha-Honor Medical Society., 59*(2), 2–10.

Granger, K. (2013). Healthcare staff must properly introduce themselves to patients. *BMJ, 347,* f5833–f5833.

Haque, O. S., & Waytz, A. (2012). Dehumanization in medicine: Causes, solutions and functions. *Perspectives on Psychological Science, 7*, 176–186.

Haslam, N. (2007). Humanising medical practice: The role of empathy. *Medical Journal of Australia, 187*(7), 381–382.

Hirshfield, L. E., & Underman, K. (2017). Empathy in medical education: A case for social construction. *Patient Education and Counseling, 100*(4), 785–787.

Howick, J., & Rees, S. (2017). Overthrowing barriers to empathy in healthcare: empathy in the age of the internet. *Journal of the Royal Society of Medicine*, 1–6.

Jeffrey, D. I. (2018). *Exploring empathy with medical students: A qualitative longitudinal phenomenological study.* (PhD), University of Edinburgh. Retrieved from https://www.pure.ed.ac.uk/admin/editor/dk/atira/pure/api/shared/model/base_uk/studentthesis/editor/studentthesiseditor.xhtml?id=59249782. Accessed 6 June 2018.

Jeffrey, D. I. (2019). *Exploring empathy with medical students.* London: Palgrave Macmillan.

Klaver, K., & Baart, A. (2016). How can attending physicians be more attentive? On being attentive versus producing attentiveness. *Medicine, Health Care, and Philosophy, 19*, 351–359.

Konner, M. (1987). *Becoming a doctor: A journey of initiation in medical school.* New York: Viking Press.

Levinas, E. (2006). *Humanism of the other.* Urbana, IL: University of Illinois Press.

Maben, J., Shuldman, C., & Taylor, C., e. a. (2017). A realist informed mixed methods evaluation of Schwartz center rounds in England. Retrieved from https://www.pointofcarefoundation.org.uk/resource/a-realist-informed-mixed-methods-evaluation-of-schwartz-center-rounds-in-england-full-report/.

Maxwell, B. (2008). *Professional ethics education: Studies in compassionate empathy.* New York: Springer.

McNaughton, N. (2013). Discourse (s) of emotion within medical education: The ever-present absence. *Medical Education, 47*(1), 71–79.

Monrouxe, L. V., & Rees, C. E. (2009). Picking up the gauntlet: Constructing medical education as a social science. *Medical Education, 43*, 196–198.

Monrouxe, L. V., Rees, C. E., & Hu, W. (2011). Differences in medical students' explicit discourses of professionalism: Acting, representing, becoming. *Medical Education, 45*(6), 585–602.

Montgomery, K. (2006). *How doctors think: Clinical judgment and the practice of medicine.* Oxford: Oxford University Press.

Nussbaum, M. (2003). *Upheavals of thought: The intelligence of emotions.* Cambridge: Cambridge University Press.

Nussbaum, M. (2013). *Creating capabiliities*. Cambridge, MA: Harvard University Press.

Point of Care Foundation. (2013). Retrieved from https://www.pointofcarefoun dation.org.uk/.

Ricoeur, P. (1992). *Oneself as another*. Chicago: University of Chicago Press.

Schafer, H. C., Helmreich, R. L., & Scheidegger, D. (1994). Human factors and safety in emergency medicine. *Resuscitation, 28,* 221–225.

Shanafelt, T., West, C., Zhao, X. H., Novotny, P., Kolars, J., Habermann, T., et al. (2005). Relationship between increased personal well-being and enhanced empathy among internal medicine residents. *Journal of General Internal Medicine, 20*(7), 559–564. https://doi.org/10.1111/j.1365-1497. 2005.0108.x.

Shapiro, J. (2008). Walking a mile in their patients' shoes: Empathy and othering in medical students' education. *Philosophy, Ethics, and Humanities in Medicine, 3,* 10–21.

Shea, S., & Lionis, C. (2014). Introducing the Journal of Compassionate Health Care. *Journal of Compassionate Health Care, 1*(1), 7.

Taylor, C., Xyrichis, A., & Leamy, M. C., e. a. (2018). Can Schwartz Center Rounds support healthcare staff with emotional challenges at work, and how do they compare with other interventions aimed at providing similar support? A systematic review and scoping reviews. *BMJ Open, 8,* e024254. http://doi. org/10.1136/bmjopen-2018-024254.

The Department of Health and Social Care. (2015). *The NHS Constitution*. Retrieved from London: https://www.gov.uk/government/publicati ons/the-nhs-constitution-for-england.

The King's Fund. (2013). *Point of care programme*. Retrieved from https:// www.kingsfund.org.uk/projects/point-of-care/about.

Underman, K., & Hirshfield, L. E. (2016). Detached concern?: Emotional social ization in twenty-first century medical education. *Social Science and Medicine, 160,* 94–101.

Warmington, S. (2012). Practising engagement: Infusing communication with empathy and compassion in medical students' clinical encounters. *Health, 16*(3), 327–342. https://doi.org/10.1177/1363459311416834.

Weatherall, D. (1994). The inhumanity of medicine. *BMJ, 309,* 1671.

INDEX